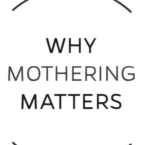

WHY
MOTHERING
MATTERS

T0161499

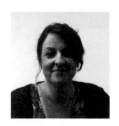

About the author

Maddie McMahon is a doula, doula course leader and breastfeeding counsellor in Cambridge, and has vast experience supporting new parents. She writes a blog about birth and breastfeeding issues at www.thebirthhub.co.uk and is the author of *Why Doulas Matter*.

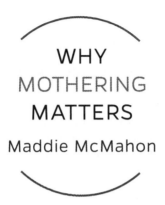

WHY
MOTHERING
MATTERS

Maddie McMahon

pinter & martin

Why Mothering Matters (Pinter & Martin Why It Matters 13)

First published by Pinter & Martin Ltd 2018

©2018 Maddie McMahon

Mothers Matter poem page 147 © Kati Edwards

Maddie McMahon has asserted her moral right to be identified as the author of this work in accordance with the Copyright, Designs and Patents Act of 1988.

ISBN 978-1-78066-590-0

Also available as an ebook

Pinter & Martin Why It Matters ISSN 2056-8657
Series editor: Susan Last
Index: Helen Bilton

British Library Cataloguing-in-Publication Data

A catalogue record for this book is available from the British Library.

Set in Minion

Printed and bound in the EU by Hussar

This book has been printed on paper that is sourced and harvested from sustainable forests and is FSC accredited.
Pinter & Martin Ltd
6 Effra Parade
London SW2 1PS
pinterandmartin.com

Contents

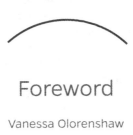

Foreword

Vanessa Olorenshaw

In *Of Woman Born*, Adrienne Rich dared to speak what I, to my shame, only truly appreciated once becoming a mother myself: that we are all born of women. We all share a fundamental experience: that our first nine months were spent held within, nurtured, fed and protected by our mothers. If this doesn't matter, then, the question must be asked, what on earth does?

As a doula, Maddie has immense experience in the rawness and power of the moment of birth, the delicate process of birthing and labour, and of the uniquely fragile and intense post-partum period. It is this experience and wisdom which shines through her book. She writes with warmth but without apology about the value of mothers and the needs of children. These are important, human, issues.

Despite my feminist leanings I had never really got it until I was in the soup of postpartum hormones and subsequently immersed in the hard graft of caring for babies and young children, harbouring the distinct feeling that I was a rather terrible feminist and had become that most despised of unfashionable creatures, known by many names: housewife; homemaker; stay at home mum; just a mum. This was despite feeling my most powerful (in birth) and needed (through breastfeeding and mothering). This was despite building a relationship with two vulnerable people to whom I was their whole world. Rather, the question struck me: 'Why is this hard work only recognised as such when someone else is paid to do it?'

Our culture insists that we 'return to normal'. That we continue as before. As though we haven't changed. There are those who insist that mothering (in philosophy and practice) can be intensely empowering and that it is our society's failure to acknowledge (let alone adequately support) mothering work that lies behind some of the manifest injustices facing women in our society. As a feminist, I have long argued that we must and should enable every woman to choose not be a mother, to choose to be a mother while also having an occupation or career outside the home, and to access free and safe reproductive services and contraception. However, we neglect the full picture, the full tapestry of motherhood, if we neglect to see the value of mothering and mothers in caring for their children.

If we are to achieve a semblance of women's liberation, a life where we are free to define our own existence, to value mothers and mothering, with the ability to live, care and love without penalty but with true support, then the barriers and penalties faced by women in the exercise of their maternity and maternal lives must be demolished. Works such as *Why Mothering Matters* will, I hope, prove to be the wrecking balls, with a nipple on the front for fun.

Vanessa Olorenshaw is a breastfeeding counsellor, feminist activist and the author of *Liberating Motherhood, Birthing the Purplestockings Movement*, published by Womancraft.

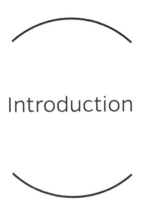

Introduction

'Motherhood is one of the most challenging and creative jobs anyone can do. The goal is to remake the world so that our choices are not so stark.'

Naomi Wolf

On the shelf next to me sits my grandmother's button box. It was her mother's before her, I think. The buttons inside are a historical record. Digging down through the layers is like archaeology; buttons and hooks from generations gone by, from clothes with stiff collars and long skirts. I think of the 'old style hats and coats' of Larkin's poem and his assertion that they 'fuck you up, your Mum and Dad'. I wonder at the hurt and pain in those words and the unrealistic simplicity of his message – 'don't have any kids yourself'.

Sometimes, as I take a button out to sew onto something, or throw my spare buttons in on top, I feel a visceral sense of connection through the generations; the old, work-roughened fingers, genetically related to mine, that have searched the depths of this box, seeking just the right size, shape and colour. Pieces of old cotton, weaving through the holes, prompt thoughts of the threads that connect us as mothers; the skills we pass down, the time spent together and alone, sewing together the frayed edges of the family, darning the holes in my soul.

Surely no one would be hard pressed to answer the question of why mothers matter? If our species is to survive, we need people to gestate, birth and nurture the next generation. But women are more than walking, talking uteruses and breasts. And the act of mothering can, and does, extend beyond women. Yes, they can '*fill you with the faults they had, and add some extra, just for you*'* but mothers can also be the universal source of unconditional love, sowing (and sewing?) the seeds of a deep sense of self-worth.

Mothering is an enormous topic: vital to life itself, of massive importance to the optimal development of children, it has an enormous impact on the psychological state of women. At this point in history, the very act of mothering seems to be under constant attack. It is also being rethought and reshaped in ways we would never have considered possible just a few generations ago.

In the original draft of my first book in this series, *Why Doulas Matter*, I wrote that the act of writing those chapters on doulas had done nothing more than impress on me once again that it is not doulas who matter, but those we serve – the people at the coalface of parenting. So I am honoured, and not a little overwhelmed, to have been given the opportunity to celebrate the millions of people out there toiling 24/7 bringing up the next generation. I hope to explore what mothering means to the world, and how the world treats mothers. I want

---

* If you don't know Larkin's poem, *This Be The Verse*, here it is: www. poetryfoundation.org/poems-and-poets/poems/detail/48419

to ask some big, eternal questions. And I want to give a voice to as many parents as I can, because it is only by listening to the lived experience of real people that we can learn how best to support them.

In many respects I am totally unqualified to write this book. I am not a sociologist or psychologist. I am not a historian or academic researcher. Yet to explore this massive topic demands something of all of those. I'm going to take a stab at it because I am, first and foremost, a mother. I am also a doula, breastfeeding counsellor, teacher, writer and passionate admirer of mothers. I have many years of mothers' voices living in my heart. I believe that mothers need to be heard and celebrated.

I have sat and watched and listened to mothers. I see that stepping through the threshold to motherhood is not something that happens in one fell swoop. We put on the robes of motherhood in layers, building up our sense of identity throughout pregnancy, birth and the early months of our baby's life. We are too often blamed and blame ourselves for everything. Becoming a mother feels more complicated and painful than ever. Without exception, we bear guilt. Motherhood, especially in the West, has become a 'damned if you do, damned if you don't' competitive battlefield. In our anxiety to get it right, we turn to the marketplace – to the legions of 'experts' and childcare manual authors who grow fat on our insecurities and doubt.

A large proportion of mothers now work full-time while still doing the majority of the childcare and domestic tasks. Around the world, the economic contribution of women means the difference between full stomachs and starvation for the majority of families. Most female work is drudging, badly paid, back-breaking, sometimes illegal and often downright dangerous.

Mothers around the world 'bring forth in suffering', not through God's will, but because, it seems, mothers must be submerged, disempowered and forgotten. Is there another way? What would happen if our bodies were celebrated for the effortless way we can bear children and feed them, instead of using our curves and breasts to sell products?

What if mothers had a voice? What if we all took back what is ours by right – our birthright – to labour and give birth safely with skilled loving attendants, in the place of our choice; to be supported with patience and loving care through the transition to parenthood; to be assisted by affordable childcare, equal pay or financial support to stay at home with our children if that is what we choose? How might it feel to fully step into our power as mothers?

What happens to a woman when she becomes a mother? The answer to that seemingly simple question has always been elusive. It seems to me that even the question is becoming more complicated. Is the physical and psychological experience of having a child the same for everyone? What influence does society and culture have on our experience of birthing and parenting? What *makes* a mother and what is the difference, if any, between the noun 'mother' and the action of 'mothering'? These are questions that interest me. You may have others. You might have some answers, too. If so, I'd love to hear them. Exploring these ideas relies on dialogue: sharing our thoughts and feelings and carving out new ways of living and loving.

Mothering is the ultimate expression of the 'personal is the political'. The 'small', the 'domestic', the minutiae of everyday life with small people can seem unimportant and not worthy of policy or social engineering. So rather than offering answers, this book's main question will be – why is this? Why are carers consistently diminished and discriminated against in our culture? Mothers and the act of mothering *matter* and I want to know why that is not a truth universally acknowledged.

A word about words

I have spent much of my time writing this book worrying about the words I use. I know the words I choose have the capacity to wound. I know the very words mothering and mother may hurt those who parent, but who do not identify with those terms. It grieves me to think that I might hurt anyone, even inadvertently. I am a mother and I care for mothers and I think mothers are amazing, powerful and important. I work with women who identify with the word mother. They are proud of owning the term and so, for them I will use it. I also believe that mothering, as a word of action, has a place beyond the narrow definition of parenthood. The caring, nurturing, modelling and mentoring elements are something anyone can do for another. I can choose to see mothering as a verb, something we do, something that enriches us and that should be celebrated, whoever is doing it. It's why doulas say we 'mother the mother'.

I subscribe to the wise counsel given by Trevor McDonald, La Leche League Leader, trans father and author of *Where's the Mother? Stories from a Transgender Dad.* He says, just 'use more words'. This simple premise sums it up for me: there are parents, there are mothers, there are fathers, there are birthing people. People use various different pronouns. When it comes to gender politics, we all identify at different points along a complex and beautiful spectrum. We are all utterly gorgeous and diverse, raising our kids as best we can. We are almost always good enough. And good enough is always absolutely, bloody awesome.

So, in an attempt to be truly inclusive, I will be talking about mothers and women in this book, but I'll also use the terms people and parents. In real life, I'd ask *you* what you want to be called, because that is simple politeness. I hope and believe that the future depends on us all listening to each other and trying to be kind. Inclusivity means accepting difference, including everyone and celebrating diversity. Feminism is about making sure we all have a voice and are treated with respect and good, old-fashioned courtesy. That is my idea of intersectional feminism.

I know I can't speak for all. I can't, in all honesty, speak for anyone except myself, a straight, white woman in 21st-century England. But I hope I can be a friend to those who are proud to be women and mothers and those who, for whatever reason, are struggling. In our beautiful, complex and ever-changing modern world there are many kinds of people embarking on parenthood, and many different kinds of people supporting them along the way.

During my years working with families I have been honoured to walk the path with all sorts of family structures. I have supported mothers and those who do not see themselves as mothers, despite birthing or parenting a child. I have come to revel in the complexities of modern families and know in my heart that it is attachment – in other words, love – that matters, not who the parents are or what they look like.

So, if you are growing a person, in your belly or out in the world, if you are a gardener of small humans: this book is for you. You are doing, quite literally, the most important job in the world. Don't be fooled into thinking bankers or chief executives or politicians are more vital; your role secures not only the future of the human race, but can also mean the difference between a future in which we merely survive or one in which we thrive.

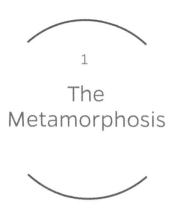

1

The
Metamorphosis

*'I cannot make you understand. I cannot make anyone
understand what is happening inside me. I cannot even
explain it to myself.'*

Franz Kafka, *The Metamorphosis*

What does it mean to become a mother?

Am I a snake, shedding my skin and revealing the mother
underneath? Did I always know how to do this? Was it always
there, waiting for expression? Is it a painful transition? Do I
need to grow before my skin splits and the mother in me can
struggle free?

Or am I a cuttlefish, changing my colours on a whim,
according to the circumstances? Effortlessly blending in with
my environment or changing to match all the other mothers?
Perhaps I'm the puffer fish, full of hot air, changing my shape
and size to appear stronger and less vulnerable.

I wonder if I am a butterfly, nestled snugly in my chrysalis,
just like a child in the womb, waiting for the changes in me

to manifest? Mutating slowly, before struggling free from the prison of who I was before. I need to pause, resting after the struggle of birth, allowing my wings to dry and unfurl before I fly.

What does it mean to become a mother? I don't know. But I do know that it is a transition; a time of transmogrification, of growth, of emotional upheaval. It is a metamorphosis of epic proportions, even if we attempt to deny those changes at first. Deeply, at the cellular level, we are being reborn.

'Yes it changed everything, but at first I was in denial about it... I look back at the person I was before I had kids and I don't recognise that person at all. Having children has taught me so much and changed me for the better in a hundred ways. It's made me less egotistical, more confident, more knowledgeable, more empathic, more patient and more accepting.' Samantha Norman

During my years as a doula, I have watched this metamorphosis play out in many ways. The change starts before pregnancy, when we idly wonder what it might feel like to be a mother. We may think of our own mothers and whether we wish to parent in a similar way. Women with mother-shaped holes in their childhoods may wonder if they will know how to be a parent. People with toxic parents may worry about passing on the hurt and despair to their own children, while others are secure in the knowledge that they will be parenting in the same way they were brought up.

Pregnancy is a time when profound changes are happening, not just in a woman's body, but in her mind. We begin to dream forward, trying on the mother-mantle for size. Everywhere we go there are mothers, and we watch and listen. We might feel happy in our circles, confident we will do things the way our sisters and mothers did. Others, however, are searching for a manual, a 'how to', to guide them through the mysteries of baby care.

It feels to me, as I watch women emerge from their chrysalises, that becoming a mother is just as much about letting go of old roles and assumptions as it is about forming new ones. The way we label ourselves and each other is caused by and perpetuates social attitudes. And becoming a mother is often seen as our one and only label. This is exemplified perfectly by the traditional man from northern England addressing his wife as 'ma' or 'mother'. Her role as nurturer and homemaker is, for him, her primary function, beyond her role as his life partner.

Yet nowhere is anyone talking about the changes in ourselves, in our very sense of identity, or supporting and guiding us as we walk the path. How does it feel to change from the woman on the Tube that men's eyes gravitate towards, to the invisible woman pushing the pram, doors swinging shut in our faces? How does it feel to be listened to and respected in a meeting at work one day, and the butt of jokes about 'baby brain' the next? How does it feel to be pregnant against your will, or looked down on for being young, single or 'different' in some way? How does it feel to realise you would lay down your life for another, in a heartbeat?

No one tells us that our brain is being reshaped, new synapses being created daily, as we learn and adapt to our new role. The hormones of motherhood create new abilities and possibilities; motherhood is love and love is a state that makes for strength and confidence. As 'mummy brain' researcher Dr Craig Kinsley from the University of Richmond in the US says:

'There's something about pregnancy and subsequent exposure to offspring that creates a more adaptive brain, one that's generally less susceptible to fear and stress.'

I have come to realise that, when a woman has a baby, especially her first, her brain is being systematically reconstructed. To all intents and purposes, we have the cognitive builders in. There is a wholesale redecoration, reorganisation and an extension being built. Women laugh, and are laughed at, because of 'baby brain', but it is much less common to crow about the fact that motherhood makes our brains more efficient and capable. The process takes a while, but eventually, once the sleep deprivation is loosening its grip and a new-normal is beginning to take shape, most mothers begin to notice real changes in their cognitive function and the way they view life, the universe and everything.

Many women can identify a massive shift in themselves that starts with the birth of their first child. As scientist-turned-birthworker Sophie Messager says, *'The way I think changed completely. I became less organised and much more creative.'*

Together with the wholesale refurbishment in the brain, there is a physical transformation during pregnancy that is obvious to the passing stranger. However, there are changes afoot that are less visible. The way women feel about those shifts is also very rarely spoken about:

'My body changed from girl to woman over night; I was a slight, flat athletic 17-year-old that summer and a curved, voluptuous woman by autumn. My breasts became swollen and beautiful and my nipples darkened and sprang out in readiness to feed my baby... in a very exciting way!' Becky Talbot

Pregnancy can bring a new-found joy in our bodies, a joy that we have been denied since we were young girls and became aware and ashamed of our female form.

'...after taking pictures of myself at 38 weeks pregnant, I saw something amazing, I felt like a ripe fruit, all the force of life blooming. I was huge and I loved it!' Lyndsey Dawn Kindred

However, growing up in a culture that puts so much emphasis on physical perfection can make pregnancy difficult for some women. Patriarchal attitudes that women should not take up too much space, not be loud and 'in your face' persist. We are celebrated for being smooth, small and blemish-free. Not all of the mothers I support here in 21st-century England feel enriched or empowered by pregnancy or motherhood. It seems our culture has a rather different view of the capabilities of a woman who is rearing children.

'Unfortunately, I hated it. The sickness and constant tiredness left me weak and unable to do much. My hair became greasy and I broke out in zits. It was worse than puberty... I no longer recognised the weak immobile lumpy body I saw in the mirror. I felt ugly.' Tracey Sealey

As Milli Hill, author of *The Positive Birth Book* and founder of the Positive Birth Movement, so eloquently explains:

'Motherhood is pathologised – used to diminish us and suggest we are weakly at the mercy of our faulty bodies. Just as the woman who asserts herself is often accused of being on her period... so pregnant women and mums find themselves called out for everyday errors, which were probably totally unrelated to their gestational status.'

The message that comes across loud and clear is that the culture I live in seems to care very little about mothers and babies. The Victorian 'angel of the hearth' image persists, and the idea of the 'good mother' still motivates us. Motherhood can still be seen as the pinnacle of a woman's achievement in life (to the extent that women who wish to remain childless are often admonished and disbelieved), but the process of reproduction and the end result, the baby, must be hidden away and not impact upon a woman's sexual and economic availability. Furthermore, the idea that all the ills of society can be laid at mothers' door has firmly taken root in our collective consciousness: reports of muggings, drug culture, poverty and unemployment are all greeted with the phrase, *'I blame the mother'*.

How much of the 'brain fog' of motherhood is self-perpetuating, I don't know. What I do know is that most of my clients have grown up in a society that takes a dim view of motherhood. As a teenager and young woman in the 1980s, my aim in life was to avoid the 'domestic servitude' of my mother's generation. At university, my Woman's Studies tutor introduced us to Betty Friedan's 'walking corpses',[1] the housewives suffering from the 'problem with no name' as they wandered through their prosaic lives weighed down by a vague sense of dissatisfaction. I couldn't think of anything worse than being pitied and patronised, surrounded by a raggle-taggle litter of snot-nosed kids hanging off my apron strings.

In my grandmother's lifetime, we moved from the image of the domestic angel instilling moral rectitude in the next generation (and boy, did my grandmother take that job seriously!) to a widespread notion that married women with children were undermining the feminist revolution. This image pervades every corner of our culture. Even now, pregnant women are often considered less able at work, passed over for promotion and manoeuvred out of the office at the earliest opportunity. It's hardly surprising we internalise this message.

It can feel very strange indeed at first, this massive change. I sometimes look at my clients and reflect on what an earthquake is happening in their lives; everything shakes and cracks and chasms can appear in their relationships, sense of self and perceptions of everything. One day we are at work, interacting with colleagues, and the next we are mooching around at home, at a loose end, an observer of life rather than a participant. After the baby is born, the social isolation can worsen. At home, in the early days, we are either ignored, our 'privacy being respected', or inundated by well-meaning visitors. It seems many of us are not considered worthy of empowering support, the kind that trusts in a mother's innate ability to parent her child and provides practical help while she finds her feet. Instead we are micromanaged, criticised, coerced and overwhelmed with well-meaning, conflicting advice. This can be especially true for mothers who may be perceived as being 'less able' than average.

'I was 15 and treated like a 3 year old... [I was] told I could not do it, I could not be a mother, I was too young, I was wasting my life, I would never amount to anything. I suffered psychologically for many years.' Nikki Mather

Doulas and midwives often remind parents that they can't eat flowers, encouraging them to think about what they actually do need. Constant calls to leave the housework and sleep when the baby sleeps don't actually provide any practical support; women have to sit on the sofa, stuck under a nursing or sleeping baby, looking at the chaos, unable to put the baby down without screams of protest. No wonder so many of us crumple under the weight of depression and anxiety.

Yet these days can also be filled with euphoria. The feeling of achievement and the small, daily pleasures our children give us are designed to keep us emotionally invested in parenting. The hormones of new motherhood, which bond us to our babies, keep us chilled, help us sleep, quickly stem the flow of postnatal bleeding, contract our wombs and continue the work of the 'brain-builders', lighting up the pleasure centres in our brains with every sniff of the baby's head or cooing conversation.

When a mother is well supported, by family, friends, neighbours and her wider community, when society values her and her work, she can leap into the parallel challenge of working out her multiple identities with aplomb. Being a mother, a lover, a sister and a daughter simultaneously is a juggle that takes a while for many of us to master with a modicum of good grace. Lactating breasts that dribble when he kisses them can be confusing or off-putting for a while. Managing a granny's memories of motherhood 20 or 30 or 40 years ago can be irritating or illuminating by turns. Deciding whether to divide loyalties between children and employer, or worse, having absolutely no financial choice, can be traumatic.

And when a woman is alone, without appropriate support, when she is perhaps dragging some heavy baggage into motherhood, this whole transition can be more difficult. Mother Nature has given us some pretty awesome superpowers, but there are internal and external barriers that sometimes prevent us from accessing the deep joy of parenting. This book is about some of those superpowers and just a few of those challenges.

> *'I was stifled by pride, but in actual fact I needed a shit load of help that I wasn't prepared to ask for.'* Ellie Cook

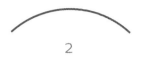

2

Mothering in a Maelstrom

'If family life and the work of care and nurture were to be valued, elevated and respected... then we would be on our way to a fairer society.'

Vanessa Olorenshaw, *Liberating Motherhood*

I'm walking around Mothercare on a spring morning. Everything is divided up into rows of pink and blue. There are complicated-looking contraptions for everything, from changing nappies to bathing baby. The list of essential items for mother and infant seems to have grown exponentially since I had my first baby in 2000. Back then, in a little book by Miriam Stoppard, I was firmly told that I needed:

- 6 baby vests
- 6 babygrows
- A cardigan
- A coat or snowsuit
- A hat
- Nappies
- Cotton wool

- A 'receiving blanket' (I had no idea what this was)
- Some muslin squares (this fascinated me, as I couldn't imagine what they might be for)
- Nappy cream
- A Moses basket with a mattress, sheets and blankets
- A car seat

Granny and her homies knitted me blankets. Cot sheets appeared from I can't remember where. Mother-in-law knitted cardigans. A Moses basket was found somewhere, second-hand, but I was reliably told he could sleep in a drawer if I didn't have one, as long as I had a decent mattress to put in it.

I bought a front-opening nightie (white – oh, how I regretted that), a nursing bra, maternity pads and mysterious-looking pads for my nipples, which my father later mistook as coasters for his coffee cup.

As I wander and wonder around the shop 16 years later, I am bewildered at the choice and the never-ending list of must-haves. I see all this 'stuff' in my clients' houses every day:

- 6-8 x sleepsuits
- 4 x wrap-over vests
- 6-8 x bodysuits
- sun hat
- 2 x soft cotton hats
- 2 x cardigans
- 2-3 x socks (pairs)
- 2 x scratch mitts (pairs)
- Weathershield
- Parasol
- Infant car seat
- Child view mirror
- Changing bag
- Cosytoe (say what?)
- Moses basket and stand or crib

- Cot or cot bed
- Mattresses
- Waterproof mattress covers
- 4 x fitted mattress sheets
- 4 x flat sheets
- 2-3 x blankets (including cotton cellular blankets)
- Changing unit or cot-top changer
- Baby listening monitor with or without a two-way speaker system or even a video camera
- Room thermometer
- Bath thermometer
- Nappy pail and lid or nappy disposal system
- 3 x nursing bras
- 2 x sleep bras
- Easy opening nightwear
- Breast pads – disposable or reusable
- 20 x muslin squares
- Breastfeeding support pillow
- Nursing tops
- Cot mobile
- Breast pump
- Breast milk storage bags
- Bottles/steriliser
- Soothers/dummies
- Nipple shields and breast shells
- Various creams, for bums and tums and nips
- A very, very expensive, fashionable (and often highly impractical) buggy or pram

A lot of these products are undeniably useful and may make our lives easier and more convenient. But I wonder what messages we are sending new parents? Do we need all this gumpf in order to be 'good' mothers? What subtle and not so subtle influences dictate what we buy and what we don't, and what kind of parents we develop into? How does it feel to be on the receiving end of this pressure to acquire 'stuff'? And how does it feel to not have the money to buy it? The power of the brand and the lure of the shiny new products can leave many feeling guilty or a failure when they can't provide their children with the 'best of everything'.

'As a new mum... I was very influenced by societal expectations, perceived norms and mainstream media... I was influenced by One Born Every Minute... *and* Supernanny *for top parenting tips... I remember my dad's shed had tools in an SMA tin so it was a profound formula brand... Pampers nappies were 'the best brand'... Terry towelling nappies were a "nightmare"'.*
Katie Olliffe

What most of us don't consider is that the foundations of how we parent are deeply rooted in our own experiences as babies and children. How resilient we are to the knocks and bumps along life's path, our emotional literacy, our responsiveness to our children's needs and feelings, all have their source in our first relationships.

Mia Scotland, clinical psychologist, told me:

'Science began to ask the question "what does a baby want" back in the 1950s, with the now famous studies of Harlow's monkeys... researchers were amazed to find that, when given a choice, baby monkeys chose cuddles over milk. The long-held belief that 'so long as baby has been changed, fed and winded, there's no reason to do anything more', is out of date. Now we need to ask 'has baby been cuddled?'

Harlow's monkeys showed us that those babies who weren't cuddled grew up to be rubbish mothers themselves. They didn't know how to care for a baby, they pushed them away. It is heart-breaking to see the videos. It seems to be the same for humans. Those of us who grew up with poor attachments are more likely to play that out in our own parenting. The difference is that humans can make decisions and plan ahead in a way that monkeys don't appear to do. So we can choose to do it differently, and enlist the help of therapists or make a conscious decision to gather loving people around us. This is best done before conception, but useful at any time in your parenting journey.'

And so it is that we bring the whole of ourselves into parenting; every relationship, life experience and media image influences our attitudes and choices. Our families often have a profound effect on these early days with a baby and how we feel about the choices we are making. Many of us will swim with the crowd, while others manage to stay true to our instinctive feelings about what is right and wrong for our children.

But when that instinct is in direct opposition to the cultural influences around us, the cognitive dissonance that can result is paralysing. My work as a doula regularly involves sitting with mothers as they desperately try to work out whose advice to listen to. Sometimes they are doing everything they can to drown out the voices inside, having so little faith in their own instincts.

'I was so lost in a chaotic and foreign world I needed my hand held constantly. I was fighting instincts as well as having them laughed at and I spiralled downwards quickly and for a long time.' Sarah Caldwell

Traditionally we have been surrounded by our extended families and the discourse would probably have been pretty consistent; the conversation about babycare and the needs of the new mother would have been rooted in history and culture. There would have been a firm connection with tradition, and with the rituals surrounding birth and parenting, giving a woman a deep sense of communion with her ancestors and a firm foundation for motherhood.

I have been musing on why this connection with traditional rituals seems more firmly rooted in some, and I think it comes from what some people call 'cultural resilience': the values, customs and rituals, our shared beliefs and cultural norms, which bind us together and enable us to deal with adversity and adapt to change. I certainly see mothers who benefit deeply from feeling a strong connection with their families and culture and feel that their traditions sing in tune with the instinctive song in their hearts and guts.

'The world around me shaped me more towards attachment parenting than anything... I found myself starting to listen to more views from my mother-in-law and places like Africa and Nepal, where babies are carried, stay with mum 24/7, feed to sleep, sleep with mum. I don't know how but I think it was something that just came from within.' Seema Barua

This resilience can mean that even when these long lines of tradition are breaking down, we can feel a strength and faith in our own intuitive parenting impulses and cope with challenges to our parenting choices. Even when everything around us tries to bend us out of shape, resilience means we can stay true to our hearts.

'I faced so much pressure from my mother-in-law to bottle feed my daughter as this was the best way to have a "healthy", i.e. fat baby. She even went as far as telling me to pop baby rusks in there, saying she did this with her own week-old babies. I was horrified... I stuck to my guns and breastfed until 20 months. There wasn't a single time she didn't express her disdain at my decision, blaming my daughter's reflux, cradle cap and dairy allergy on the fact that I didn't bottle feed her.' Anon

I think we need to work hard to help mothers to maintain

this resilience. An internal faith or deeply embedded sense of tradition and ritual can protect against depression, isolation and low self-esteem. Practical abilities passed down from one mum to the next help us face the everyday tasks of mothering. And a sense of fellowship within a network of neighbours and friends provides social cohesion, support and solidarity.

'Second time around, five years later with a different partner and a different life, I found my tribe. A big group of APers ['attachment parenting' – a philosophy centred around minimising any separation of mother and baby] *and I felt like I was home! I was supported and I found peace with my parenting style and my natural ability. A complete 180 but it was needed as it fixed me.'* Sarah Caldwell

This sense of camaraderie with a group sharing similar experiences has all but disappeared for many women in the UK. They are often isolated from family by geography or relationship breakdown, have few friends with children or have much older parents who can't be of practical help. We are having to reinvent support structures from scratch. These new ways of building cultural resilience can have a profound impact on a woman's journey. Support groups, both face-to-face and on social media, are slowly bringing back a sense of community. These groups are often a source of ideas, a place to share and pay forward the help you received. They are also beginning to become a receptacle of remembering and protecting ancient knowledge and ritual; of reintroducing us to our past and creating our own, newly-minted, rituals for ourselves and our children.

Doula Sophie Messager is passionate about reclaiming tradition and creating a renaissance in ritual and ceremony around the childbearing year. She brings like-minded women together in a popular and growing Facebook group. As she puts it:

'I started this group because I feel that something is really missing in our culture when it comes to supporting pregnant, birthing and new mothers. They need to feel nurtured physically, emotionally and spiritually. We used to have this in the West, but we simply have lost the way.'

We need to work hard to protect these groups; to nurture, support and help them grow. It is so important that the new social structures we are creating are inclusive so that all can access the sense of community they create. However old, whatever colour or gender we are, there should be a place for us to meet, feel loved, unconditionally accepted and held as we grow into our mothering identity. And we just know when we've found our kindred spirits:

'...you can be yourself with them, like friends you've known forever even if you've only just met.' Charlotte Ashley-Roberts

'without the support of local breastfeeding peer supporters at baby cafés and seeing women feeding out and about/posting brelfies [breastfeeding selfies] *I think I would be much more limited in my ability to feed up to a year.'* Kasiaa Rees

Everywhere I go, parents are reaching out, looking for connections and support. It seems a great shame that the single biggest move to create more face-to-face support for parents in the UK since the inception of the NHS – Children's Centres – are now being systematically dismantled for no good reason. In an age of austerity, investing in the 0–3 age group is proven to save society money and resources. Yet the kind of support on offer to parents can vary wildly around the country and opinions about what does, and doesn't, constitute good support are passionately debated. What is not up for debate is the solid evidence that creating the conditions for secure attachment between parents and children builds resilient, healthy families.

And children from such families typically grow into resourceful, strong, emotionally stable adults who will parent effectively in their turn.

Of course, social isolation or the lack of a clan of like-minded friends doesn't always result in negative experiences. Sometimes the opportunity to start from scratch, to make it up as we go along, can be very fulfilling and supportive of our self-esteem.

'I'm not close to my mum. She was an abusive alcoholic throughout my childhood and she did a lot of things that disconnected us and made me lose respect for her. In terms of mothering I feel somewhat "without roots" and as sad as that may seem, it's quite liberating – I'm making up my own rules, paving my own path and embracing every step.' Anon

'I was the first of all my friends to marry and have kids (by about 10 years!) so I was winging it from the start. The beauty of that was that I seemed like a great mum as I had nobody to compare myself to!' Lauren Mishcon

'At first I felt like I was falling down a black hole, every day being on my own. I had friends but no practical help and it was hard, very hard. However, reflecting back I feel this early experience has given me a firm foundation for both of us as parents, who we want to be and how we want to parent with limited influence or even, dare I say it, "pressure" from others around us.' Clare Cogan

But are any of us parenting in isolation? What influences are whispering in our ears, even without us realising it? I remember having a nagging feeling that everything I did was second best. I wasn't proud of my bargain hunting and make-do-and-mend lifestyle; I was ashamed of being poor and felt sad and mad every time I opened a magazine or catalogue, visited a shop or attended a baby group. The *things* people had! Yet there were moments of clarity. Times when the here and now would fall away and I was connected to all mothers everywhere, in time and space. This had first happened to me in the birth room, in late labour, and then, with a new baby, I somehow knew how to sense his mood, calm his frayed nerves and nurture him at my breast despite having no one to teach me. This instinctive 'knowing' is something many mothers report.

> *'I've never been one for dancing or singing before kids but it came out of me with my babies. A collective memory of women, to sway and rock when our babies are inside as well as out. And to soothe them with a song. Some of my most precious memories are moments I've had alone, swaying a giant belly, singing to it in the bath, or breathing in a tiny newborn that's tree-frogged up on my shoulder... These are the rituals [that] brought us a lot of joy.'* Mandy

Before I knew anything about breastfeeding, I did it to save money and was thus rather ashamed of admitting it. I became even more secretive when it became clear that neither I, nor my children, appeared to know how to wean. The adverts on the TV told me I could choose to move on. I didn't really know what that meant, but it looked a sunny place to be and seemed to involve bottles. So I bought one. My baby had other ideas! In an age before social media, I was alone and lonely, but the insidious reach of commercial influences had a profound effect on my perception of myself as a mother, as a woman and as a person.

It wasn't until I had my second child and became a doula that I began to make sense of this incessant comparing that mothers seem to do. Of course, it's a natural human trait to be constantly – consciously or unconsciously – making comparisons: 'her dress is more expensive than mine', 'his car is the next model up', 'she is thinner, prettier, more attractive than me'. Most of us allow these fleeting thoughts to pass away unnoticed without causing damage. But at times of vulnerability, when our emotional resources are depleted, these negative thoughts can be damaging.

Psychologist Katie Newns gave me some clarity on this:

'There are two ways of tending with social comparison – comparing yourself with people who are better (upward) or worse (downward). Highly motivated people tend to compare upward – assuming they are as good as or equal to the best. Someone who is not motivated or who is unhappy will tend to engage in downward comparison (in an effort to feel better about themselves). Studies have shown that frequent social comparisons have a 'dark side', with envy, guilt, regret, defensiveness, and poor job satisfaction (White et al. 2006).'

When working with new mothers it is very common for them to apologise for the state of their houses, make disparaging remarks about their own postpartum bodies and compare themselves negatively to other mothers they meet. I go to great lengths to help them kick this negative habit. Your house is more untidy than some, but much better than others (you should see mine, and I don't have the excuse of a baby!). Your postpartum belly is nature's feeding pillow, a soft cushion for a toddler's head. And those mums with their lippy on in a painted-on smile? That aura of perfection is all too often just an illusion.

As Vanessa Olorenshaw, author of *Liberating Motherhood*, notes:

'It is an injustice, cleverly camouflaged, that the work of mothers can be sabotaged by society, or blighted by hurdles they face financially and socially, and yet mothers get the blame.'

There are people out there who make an awful lot of money from this natural propensity for comparison and our understandable feelings of defensiveness and vulnerability after having a baby. We crave acceptance and are desperately looking for community. There are those who wish to push you to identify with a certain group by creating the illusion that others are judging your choices. When companies promote the idea that breastfeeding mothers are judging formula feeders, or babywearers hate pram-pushers, people are grouped behind battle lines and we become loyal to companies, rather than to each other.

'A better approach would be to exercise mindful parenting: being present in the moment and focussing on self-awareness, embracing the knowledge that parenting can be difficult, complex, and that no one can be the perfect parent.' Katie Newns, psychologist

That media and advertising can have a toxic and insidious effect on our sense of self and our interactions with others is a well-researched truth. I entreat you to resist it; mothers have more in common with each other than differences. And there is too big a battle for basic maternal and parental rights to be distracted by petty fights.

These pressures on mothers can be immense, and these days the influences are with us 24/7 in the guise of social media – a noisy place full of conflicting advice and playground pressure to 'join the in crowd'. While some of us are able to be resistant to all this and be confident and happy in our own choices, others spiral down into a very dark place if they are isolated from psychosocial support.

Self-esteem and resilience are basic human traits that are built through community, ritual, fellowship, solidarity and faith-systems. When these ingredients are missing, the new identity of mother can shake us to our core.

Katie Newns again:

'A recent study[2] found that early attachment relationships act as a prototype for all intimate relationships – including one's relationship with one's own child. How a mother conceptualises their own mother-child attachment history exerts a substantial influence over her own interactions with her child.

Further studies have supported Bowlby's theory, that internal working models of attachment tend to be perpetuated across generations. This indicates that caregivers' attitudes towards attachment may be derived from their own childhood experiences of attachment.' [3]

That patterns, vulnerabilities and behaviours can cascade down the generations seems like a no-brainer, right? I know that many mothers know this instinctively:

'Self esteem played a big part for me. Not having the confidence in my own abilities was crippling. A gift from my upbringing for sure!' Emma Kenny

Modern mothers, at least many that I meet, are like animals who have been bred in captivity. Without their herd, they flounder. We have replaced kith, kin and clan with doctors and parenting 'experts'. Our first thought, on finding we are pregnant, is to visit the doctor. Attempts to encourage women to book in directly with a midwife seem to be continuously thwarted, by GP receptionists, by women who feel that only a doctor can confirm their pregnancy and by society at large, which perpetuates the idea that pregnancy is an illness.

Instead of meeting a midwife with whom she can begin to build a relationship, a warm, understanding care-giver who will join her in celebrating, or empathise with her worries, pregnant people are all too often placed on a medical conveyor belt. They are measured and palpated, asked questions. Forms are filled in. Paperwork is completed and computerised records updated. While the numbers and checking and medical surveillance undeniably make for a safer pregnancy, there is a lack, something missing, that many women don't even realise they are craving. There is a nagging feeling that there is a gaping spiritual hole in their care.

What has struck me deeply as I work with parents is the concordance between the emotional needs of a mother and what the research tells us leads to the safest, most satisfying outcomes. For example, continuity of care, from a midwife that the mother gets to know and trust, has been shown, time and again, to be the safest form of care. Why might this be? I think most pregnant people would find it easy to answer that question. It is certainly an obvious truth for midwife Siobhan Taylor:

> 'Continuity of care and carer nurtures the woman, giving her the confidence needed to optimise her birth experience. For the midwife it gives job satisfaction, returning the role of midwife to a fulfilling vocation rather than just a job! ... The relationship built between a woman and her family and the midwife is the foundation of safe care.'

When a mother is seen by a different midwife or doctor each time during pregnancy, medical signals that all is not well can be missed. The trust and confidentiality needed for disclosures of domestic violence, abuse or mental health worries can be missing. All this is crucial. And for me, the most common symptom of lack of continuity is the gaping hole where labour care from a known and trusted caregiver should be.* Why is this so important?

---

* At the time of writing these 'trusted partnerships' between truly independent midwives and the mothers who choose them are under threat. The human right to choose where and with whom to give birth

Because the hormones of labour flow best in an environment of love, trust and safety. The warmth of unconditional approval and loving touch quite literally helps babies come out quickly and safely. As midwife Rosanne Payne explains:

> 'During labour, mutual trust between the woman and her midwife is the anchor that enables the woman to let go and her midwife to let her go. Continuity of carer during pregnancy is fundamental to the development of these trusting partnerships.'

Yet for so many women the medical pathway during pregnancy primes them for a cascade of medical intervention during birth. Every time we see a midwife in pregnancy we are asked to 'pop up onto the bed', instilling in us the habits that persist when we arrive in the labour ward; climbing into bed like poorly little girls, waiting patiently for the nice doctor to make us all better.

I am far from the media-spun stereotype of the natural birth freak – medical intervention in birth can be a Good Thing. It saves lives and for some women is a physical or psychological necessity. But medicalising birth not only sometimes leads to less-safe outcomes for mothers and babies – physical damage to mothers and babies is proven to happen at higher rates in obstetric units – it can also result in women feeling traumatised and violated by the feeling of loss of control on the conveyor belt of medical intervention.

When we come out of birth feeling hopeless and helpless we are starting motherhood from a place of depletion. Our mothering has shaky foundations. Some will spiral down into depression or anxiety. A few will suffer post-traumatic stress, stuck in the moment of extreme fear or threat, with the story playing in a loop

is at risk of being obliterated. To join the campaign to #savethemidwife, visit www.imuk.org.uk/news/judicial-review-to-protect-independent-midwifery-begins

in front of their inner eye. Many go forward into their mothering with an undermined sense of their own autonomy and strength as parents, their instinctive voice muted.

And it's not just mothers who can be traumatised by birth. Fathers and partners can carry the burden of traumatic stress into their parenting journey, affecting the dynamic and relationships within the family.

Instead of trusting the back of their hand on their child's forehead, the digital thermometer becomes essential. Instead of taking off some clothes and nursing the baby skin-to-skin, the baby is dosed up on infant paracetamol. The doctor is called and pressurised to prescribe for every normal ailment of childhood. Instead of bolstering parents' faith in their own abilities, we are medicalising the whole story.

In a capitalist, consumerist society we are sold the idea that the ancient challenges of birth and mothering are best solved by 'things': shopping lists, machines that go ping, technology and pharmaceuticals. While being a Luddite never got anyone anywhere, isn't it time to wonder whether we're throwing the baby out with the bathwater?

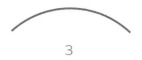

3

The Chemical Soup
of Motherhood

'When you are a mother, you are never really alone in your thoughts. A mother always has to think twice, once for herself and once for her child.'

Sophia Loren

I have been formed by a culture that taught me that the private, domestic sphere is somehow not important, somehow not *real* or as valued as public life. The first minutes, hours and days of motherhood are an unseen, intense experience that is so veiled and hidden that it is rare that a mother is emotionally prepared for it. But the enormous complexity and the beautiful perfection of this time leaves me breathless.

The more women I see welcome their babies, and the more I learn about this sacred period, the more I see it like music: a symphony unfolding, building to a crescendo, with all the instruments playing in harmony. It is an incredibly complicated piece of music, gaining in volume and intensity as she gets ready to birth. Every hour, every day, moulding and sculpting her baby to fit through her pelvis, readying the infant's body for life outside. It is a work of art in the making.

Many of the musical instruments are hormones; their tones completely distinct and their roles diverse. Together they make the sweet harmonies necessary to drive her through the birthing process. Her womb tightens, helping to move her baby around and down. The tightenings increase her hormones and so the refrain repeats, each cycle building on the last and introducing harmonious variations. Each chorus of hormone surges has an effect on her brain as well as her body; opening her mind, her womb, her bones and her heart, readying her to meet her baby.

The baby is fed by her mother's body; rich, oxygenated blood, nutrients and even good bacteria are sent baby-side. As the baby travels through the vagina, even more bacteria 'seed' the baby – forming the beginnings of the microbiome that colonises all humans and forms our immune system. We are more bacteria than human: a symbiosis of interdependent creatures making music together.

As the baby navigates through the pelvis, twisting and wriggling their way out, the rhapsody is building to a crescendo. The mother's voice may lift as she sways and writhes to the waves of energy inside her. As the widest part of the baby's head stretches the opening to her vagina to its extreme, the hormone oxytocin plays a louder note than ever before. The music is up tempo; she pants like a dog on a hot day, slowing the advancing head. And then suddenly, there is a face, a child. There is a moment, a pause in the music; all the players hold their breath for a few beats. The world stops. The child is between worlds, eyes often wide, peering into the unknown like a scuba-diver exploring an alien world. And as the last twist in the dance plays out, the baby is fully born, everyone exhales and the music starts again.

As the mother cradles her newborn, still connected to her by a rope of throbbing blood, the music is quieter, lilting and unbelievably beautiful. The hormonal notes soar unfettered. Mother and baby are suddenly wide awake and dancing together, fixated on each other's faces. The feel of the other's body, and the loving gaze as eye meets eye, making the music swell, causing her to womb to work hard again to expel the placenta. Ancient instincts move the baby to seek the breast; finding the way with the aid of scent, sight and touch. Oh, how loud the music must be for the baby, every nerve-ending jangling, every sensation completely new. Finally, upon reaching the breast and drinking deeply – a bizarre kind of new-old memory; a tune that feels vaguely familiar. It smells and tastes like home.

Oxytocin helped the mother birth her baby, it helps her milk flow and, as she bathes in the maternal music, it causes her to fall in love. Like the tiger and the elephant and the mouse mamas, the tune she dances to ensures the baby is the most beautiful thing she has ever seen. She is hyper-alert, yet simultaneously in a haze of love, as she caresses the soft skin of her newborn and scans the horizon for danger.

'In new moms, there are changes in many of the brain areas. Growth in brain regions involved in emotion regulation, empathy-related regions, but also what we call maternal motivation... In animals and humans during the postpartum period, there's an enormous desire to take care of their own child.' Pilyoung Kim, maternal brain researcher

Whether the concerto plays out without intervention or takes a longer or more complex medical route, the music is always trying to follow the same melody. Every hormonal note is slowly or quickly bonding mother and child, melding them together in a warm, sweet, fog of love. Babies born with instruments or by caesarean, or with drugs in their systems, and mothers who have other impediments to bonding with their babies, all benefit from the harmonious hormones of skin-to-skin cuddles. Babies in special care units grow more quickly and go home sooner if kept prone on their mother's chest.

Those not in the know think that one has become two. But motherbaby is still a unit, fixated on each other, interdependent and unable to truly function without the other in close proximity. The process of birth melts us, turns us to butter, softening the cervix and pelvic floor to let the baby slip out. Once the baby is earthside, he can nestle in his new habitat, the warm soft nest of his mother's arms and chest. As she cradles, nurtures and nourishes the baby with her body, she melts even more, surrendering to motherhood and the new rhythms of life with a baby. Becoming a mother, in terms of brain chemistry, looks very much like falling in love.

We are more mammal than human at this time, I think. The baby is moulding our brain; quite literally changing us into a mother with every feed and nappy change. Every hour that passes creates new synapses in the mother's brain, new connections, new abilities and moments of insight. The smell of her child lights up the reward centres in her brain. Her neocortex is sleepy, but her limbic system is working overtime, keeping her alert to danger.

Interestingly, researchers have found that while there are similar chemical changes in a man's brain when he is deeply involved in parenting, his behaviour is chiefly driven by a cognitive function that develops later in life. A woman's brain, however, plays out a brain-hormone behaviour-dance that has been there all her life. In other words, the foundations of a woman's mothering behaviour were already in her brain – proof of that old homily; 'the knowing how to mother is already inside you'. Yet a baby has such a powerful effect on the brain that male homosexual parents and fathers who provide much of the day-to-day babycare soon show the same cognitive changes – it just takes a little longer. I was once told that when we have a child, a new room opens in our hearts; a place for that child to live. Science is discovering that the room was always there, a secret door waiting to be opened – our very own, personal Narnia.

This little creature is so small and vulnerable. Without a shell, spines or sharp claws, a human baby has evolved to expect the constant close protective presence of a caregiver. Only a parent will truly do, and often only the mother, as babies instinctively know how emotionally invested they are in keeping them safe. But the strong, gentle arms of any loving human may be acceptable, at least for a while. Every attempt at putting the baby down will inevitably lead to wails of objection to the separation.

I love watching new parents find ways to placate and comfort their offspring. I see fathers walking around the house with a baby draped over their forearm, mothers working out how to tie a sling and get baby comfy in it to sleep. Lullabies are sung while rocking, patting, shhh-ing; recreating the environment of the womb for this still-foetus-like little person.

'...skin brushing skin, nuzzling and tenderly holding... the most simple acts of human relationship; the very beginning of someone's life – filled with unspoken promises of intimacy and trust. I once witnessed loving new parents take 20 mins to change a nappy and dress their baby girl as every finger and toe and every bit in between was carefully considered, uncovered and recovered. That feeling of celebration of the small things: look we dressed her/him, fed them, rocked them to sleep, carried them in the sling and it worked...' Suzanne Howlett, doula

As a mother masters new skills, her dopamine levels increase, rewarding her with a pleasurable sense of achievement. Close contact – carrying, wearing and feeding her baby – increases oxytocin and prolactin levels, increasing her milk supply, deflating her womb, slowing her bleeding and helping her sleep and wake in rhythm with the baby.

Social support networks are vital at this time. The neighbours and friends dropping by with food. The family members taking up the burden of housework and other chores. The mother's time is freed up to recover physically from the pregnancy and birth and listen to the beat of this new music that is motherhood. The high note in this tune is serotonin, levels of which are boosted by social contact, making her happier and guarding against the depression that can set in with social isolation. Surrounded by kindly helpers, who come without judgment into this sacred postpartum space, she can work her way through this psychological transition.

In many cultures this pause, this time away from normal life, is religiously observed for one lunar month. It is a 'babymoon' – a time for a new relationship to be celebrated, new rituals to be started, a special transition to be respected and honoured. Just like the honeymoon, a babymoon is time out from life after the special day, a time to stare into a lover's eyes and learn how much you mean to each other. It is also a time to step into a new role and try it on for size. The world gives us a little time and privacy to take things slowly; to figure things out for ourselves. Whether you are a birth parent or not, bathing in the hormone of love for a while, and having your friends and family support and celebrate your transition to parenthood, is, I think, your right. And it is certainly our responsibility as a society to mark these precious moments and officially approve of the laudable work of parenting. Without it, these vital roles can be overlooked and we can forget to accommodate the needs of families when we design public services.

Behind closed doors, in dark bedrooms and untidy

kitchens, in shacks and mansions, all over the world, women are morphing into mothers, people are birthing themselves as parents. And it is the baby that moulds us, sculpting the woman into the mother, the person into parent. As mother-of-two Lorette Michallon says, she wishes she'd known that her *'brain would rewire and I would birth a new version of myself.'*

As with any sculpture, the material needs to be soft. A kind of melting, relaxing or softening into mothering is what seems to happen once the excitement of the birth is over. The sweetness of the babymoon is there to allow a deep communion between the baby and her parents. The communication is two-way; they are learning each other's language, learning to love. Each time she calms her baby, each time she earns a smile or the baby turns towards her at the sound of her voice, her brain is flooded with dopamine, the brain-drug of reward. Quite literally, our babies bribe us to care for them! The system works the other way, too. The baby is rewarded by the soothing cuddles, the warm milk and the enticing sound of a parent's voice.

And so the bond is built. The love blossoms and the baby births the mother. She ripens, hanging heavy and fecund on the tree of motherhood, nourishing her baby and in turn being nourished by the joy her baby brings her.

'Research suggests that cuddling triggers a natural response that incorporates the whole nervous system, hormonal system, neural system, immune system, digestive system and so on. Cuddling stimulates calm, relaxation, love, and all sorts of good healthy things in the body, such as healthy digestion and immune system functioning. And it is best done skin-to-skin. There's a reason that hospitals advocate an hour of skin-to-skin when baby has been born. It's not because they like to do feel-good nicey nicey things. It's because science shows us unequivocally that it sets the baby and mother up for a better

start, and that this better start literally lasts a lifetime. Indeed, research also suggests that it may last across more than one generation. And it's true for fathers too. Skin-to-skin after birth between father and baby has been shown to strengthen the bond between them, a bond that contributes to the all-round health and vitality that lasts into the baby's future.' Mia Scotland, clinical psychologist

This chemical soup of motherhood continues through pregnancy and into nurturing and feeding the baby. The hormones of breastfeeding further add to the lullaby music of the postpartum. Prolactin and oxytocin tell the body to make and deliver milk. As the child nurses, more oxytocin floods her brain, giving her a sense of calm and connection, and, in a positive feedback loop, the tune is repeated, telling her body to make and exude more hormones and thus more milk.

Breastmilk is a veritable smorgasbord of creative chemicals – after all, breastmilk is a fluid that millions of years of evolution has perfected. Even before the baby is born, a mother's breasts are beginning to produce colostrum, the first super-food, designed specifically to protect our extremely vulnerable newborn infants. Low in fat but packed with carbs, protein and immune-supporting factors, it is easily digested and comes in small amounts – perfect for a newborn just learning to suckle who might be overwhelmed by larger volumes. It is more medicine than food; coating the gut walls, it prevents alien substances from reaching the bloodstream. It also acts as a laxative – making sure the baby expels those first sticky, black meconium poos.

With soft breasts in the first few days, mother and baby can practice the skill of breastfeeding without hard, heavy boobs making it challenging. Small amounts, regularly, guard against dehydration and the carbohydrate maintains the baby's sugar levels, giving them energy to wake and crawl to the breast for the next feed. Each time the baby latches on, the next phase in the saga is brought one step closer: the process that started with the birth of the placenta causes pregnancy hormones to diminish and the hormones of lactation to soar. All this culminates a few days in: baby has successfully 'called in the milk', resulting in warm, full, throbbing breasts and, more often than not, hot tears on the mother's cheeks.

This mature milk is low in fat compared to most mammals. Humans are designed to live on our mother's body, feeding very frequently. All primates are 'carrying species', supping on milk at short intervals and growing in size slowly. Humans have the slowest-growing babies of all, with the longest childhoods, so our milk is perfectly made to support this process. What does grow fast in human babies, however, is the brain. Fuelled by high levels of lactose sugars – the special carbohydrate in mammalian milk that is easily converted into glucose – as well as omega-3 and -6 fatty acids, babies' brains grow in size by 1% a day, nearly 65% in three months. Even more incredibly, the cerebellum, the area of the brain that is involved in movement, doubles in size in 90 days.[5]

The hormones that produce and deliver the milk, prolactin and oxytocin, guard against depression, deepen attachment, promote restful sleep and create circadian rhythms. Of course, the baby is not always born under the steam of just the mother's hormones. Increasingly, around the world, birthing people are given artificial hormones to induce or augment the process. Syntocinon, as it is known in the UK (pitocin in the US), is the artificial form of our own oxytocin and generally does a good job of creating uterine contractions and therefore dilating a mother's cervix. However, unlike its natural counterpart, syntocinon cannot cross over into the brain and create the unique conditions necessary for labour to play out in the complex way evolution has designed. It does not lead to the creation of endorphins, nature's own painkillers, resulting in more women requesting epidurals. Nor does it result in the loved up, chilled out, meditative state that oxytocin normally induces. Further, it blocks natural oxytocin production and may continue suppressing natural oxytocin long after the syntocinon has been discontinued.

The potential knock on effects of this, and other drugs used during childbirth, on breastfeeding are only just being recognised. There is evidence that interventions in labour account for some of the cases where mothers wish to breastfeed, but find it impossible or incredibly challenging. The good news is that, if you want to breastfeed, understanding the basic mechanisms of oxytocin and prolactin will probably help you: keep your baby skin-to-skin in a dim, warm environment. Put the baby to the breast or, if that is not possible, hand express colostrum regularly and feed that to the baby. Avoid filling the baby with large volumes of formula milk, which may result in a baby that is sleepy and less likely to latch on. Try to stay calm, and if adrenaline spirals out of control, have a good scream and discharge it – trying to keep a lid on it just causes it to build even more! Spend time getting to know your baby and hanging out with loved ones – and make sure they bring you your favourite food. Get some skilled, qualified breastfeeding support.[6] Find ways to catch forty winks when you can. Consider wearing your baby in a sling. Lastly and most importantly, let yourself off the hook; your birth was as it was. It certainly wasn't your fault. You did what you needed to do to get your baby out and you made the decisions you did with the information you had at the time. You are amazing.

Once those early days of learning to feed are past, we begin to realise that milk is about so much more than food. Breastfeeding is a relationship; a way to nurture as well as nourish a child. On one level, it seems to work to just take our milk for granted, using our breasts as mothering tools as we get on with the busy-ness of life. Yet our growing understanding of the magic ingredients of breastmilk is undeniably fascinating. There are chemicals that make babies feel full and sleepy and regulate appetite. There are growth factors, including peptide growth factors, and cytokines, which help cells communicate and activate the immune system. Epidermal growth factor and insulin-like growth factor are two of the other stars of the show. There are stem cells and HAMLET cells, which appear to guard against cancer. There are probiotics and oligosaccharides, which cannot be digested by the baby, but are especially designed to feed good bacteria. Then, of course, there are all the vitamins, minerals and micronutrients of every kind, changing and adapting on a daily basis to meet the needs of the child, together with ingredients that actually help a baby use these nutrients. In other words, the vitamins and minerals in breastmilk are what the scientists call 'bio-available' – easily digested and absorbed into the bloodstream and used for all the jobs of growth and development they are destined for. And all this, delivered instantly, at the right temperature, without work or preparation and needing only a few hundred calories of energy a day for the mother to produce. A high quality, energy-efficient, eco-friendly system of nutrition and health care that is unrivalled.

And what about those antibodies? Everyone knows that breastmilk contains them. Not many people stop to think about what that might actually mean. When a foetus is in her mother's womb, she receives antibodies through the placenta – from her mother and grandmother and so on back up through the maternal line. It is a true family inheritance: a baby is born with a protective shield passed down through the generations. But a newborn baby's immune system at birth is a project that is only just beginning. It will not be complete until well after the child has started primary school. Small humans are designed to rely on the microbiota – the good bacteria they get from their immediate family and the antibodies in breastmilk.

As the baby begins to nurse, she is protected in real time by the production of IgA antibodies in the milk. If a mother is sneezed over on the bus, she will make the antibodies to that particular virus and pass them to the baby, possibly as quickly as the next feed. If a mother and child are separated, and the baby or child is infected, she will return to her mother and do all she can to infect her with the same virus. Those little hands will search out her mother's face and her mother will playfully suck those chubby little fingers or toes. The virus can even enter the mother's body directly, via the child's saliva, up and into the breast via the milk ducts, affectionately and rather disgustingly called 'baby spit backwash'[7] by breastfeeding researchers. Thus, the baby communicates her needs, and the mother's body samples the attacking microbes, creates the perfect defence, and delivers it seamlessly back to the child.

There are myriad other ingredients in the chemical soup. How about those famous pheromones, a means of chemical communication that starts in the womb? Before birth, mother and baby are having a conversation, sending pheromones back and forth. These chemical signals survive the birth process, enabling a mother to recognise her own child. And by the time a baby is born, they have spent many months becoming familiar with the mother's pheromone cocktail. The baby is therefore helped to find the breast by alluring pheromone signals and is able to recognise the mother within hours of birth.

Not only do pheromones help mother and baby identify each other, but exposure to these chemicals from the mother's armpits and, through breastfeeding, from her nipples and areolas, also begins the process of sculpting a baby's brain. The pheromones and odours a baby experiences are thought to influence their later choice of partner. How strange to think you may smell like your partner's mother!

Next come good bacteria that began to colonise the baby in utero, via the birth canal and then, after birth, via the warm mother's skin and milk. The close cuddles of skin-to-skin contact and the baby nursing in the hours, days and weeks after birth are what protect the baby and begin the long process of immune system growth. The father's skin is a rich source of good bacteria too. The important thing, according to researchers, is that the baby is colonised by bacteria from their immediate family, not hospital staff or strangers.

At birth, after a moment to catch her breath and come back to herself, a mother will look, touch and then gather her baby in her arms.

'Everything around us melted away, it was just me and him and overwhelming love. The empty space inside me suddenly felt full as we instantly connected, and that feeling has never disappeared.' Ellie Longbone

If the mother and baby are separated at birth, the chemical soup has different ingredients. The bacterial diversity of the baby's skin and gut will be affected and the emotional state of parents will be different, too:

'I didn't have immediate skin-to-skin with the third – I truly believe that affected my bonding process. I felt deprived of that sense of euphoria I had experienced with the first two.' Casey

The power of early cuddles is tangible and can protect the mother from residual feelings of trauma:

'After a traumatic labour ending in an emergency caesarean, immediate skin-to-skin and an uninterrupted golden hour with my baby pulled me back from the edge. It made a huge

difference to how I felt about that birth. It also meant that breastfeeding and bonding got off to a flying start.' Tracy

As the baby lies curled between the mother's breasts in skin-to-skin contact, she acts as an incubator. If the baby is too cold, her body quickly sends hot blood to her chest, warming her baby. If baby is too hot, her chest cools down in response. This process is more responsive and accurate than any man-made incubator and does the added job of regulating the baby's heart rate and respiration. Both mother and baby are awash with oxytocin, ensuring they are both super-relaxed. This calm, warm state can create just the right environment for their instincts to kick in, so however the baby was born, and however stressed they might both have been, these skin-to-skin cuddles can push the reset button, allowing the baby to latch and drink and motherbaby to fall in love.

As mother and child lie together, hot, damp and euphoric after the throes of birth, chimeric cells from the baby are working their way through the mother's body. They may eventually work their way to her brain. An actual piece of her child may reside in her brain forever, affecting the workings of her mind. On a very real level, her child's cells help to morph her into the person she is becoming, shaping her butterfly wings as she readies herself to break free from the chrysalis.

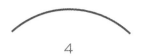

4

Hurdles and Hoops, Holding us Back

'Humanizing birth means understanding that the woman giving birth is a human being, not a machine and not just a container for making babies. Showing women – half of all people – that they are inferior and inadequate by taking away their power to give birth is a tragedy for all society.'

Marsden Wagner

This morning I sat in my garden and talked to a woman who had lost her job because her boss said she couldn't come back to work as a breastfeeding mother. I have met women who have escaped war-torn countries, walking thousands of miles, carrying their children.

Just miles from where you may be reading this book, refugee mothers are struggling to care for themselves and their children.

"'Boat bad, boat very bad". She then proceeded to explain in very broken English that they had been on the boat for seven days; "I was sick, very sick with headaches all the way". They

had been given no food, just water.' Linda Robinson MBE

I have supported women who are HIV positive being told they can't breastfeed their babies.* There is more than one woman in my life right now who is hiding from an abusive partner, trying to explain to her kids why they have run away. I have held women in my arms as they sob and tell me stories of birth trauma that has left them with the same symptoms that plague soldiers returning from war or physical scars that torment them for years, without hope of a cure.

I have talked to women about rape, female genital mutilation, domestic violence, obstetric violence, mental illness, unwanted pregnancies, access to birth control and abortion.

It is against landscapes like this that so many women are becoming mothers. It seems everywhere we go we are required to jump over hurdles and through hoops. We are held back by judgement, arbitrary rules or flagrant disregard of our human rights. Around the world, as you read this, mothers are birthing alone or without trained attendants. They are feeding their babies, despite worries about the quality or quantity of their milk. They are keeping hearth and home together, sending their children to school, counting the pennies to make sure the family is fed, hatching cunning plans to ensure clothes are clean and feet can be shod while the very fabric of society falls apart around them. While the men run around with guns, or sit in plush offices playing the game of chess that is war or big business (sometimes I wonder which is which), women keep the world turning. Despite everything, it is the mothers who hold the edges together, against all the odds of poverty, war, rape, torture: they grit their teeth and

---

* Not true, by the way. New evidence suggests HIV+ women can exclusively breastfeed, which minimises the chance of vertical transmission. See www. who.int/bulletin/volumes/88/1/10-030110/en

carry on. More than carry on; they dance and sing and sew up the holes, making and mending in direct opposition to those who would destroy.

Men suffer too, of course. Their suffering is often a direct result of the impositions and discrimination imposed on women. They are our sons, our partners, our fathers and uncles. Their pain is ours and vice-versa. This book is not about erasing the challenges facing other groups of people. We are all interconnected. Life is not a competition for the greatest victimhood and most certainly, just because we focus on a victim group it does not mean we are accusing all those not in that group of being perpetrators. In other words, my husband does not need to remind me that not all men are rapists, just because I have been the victim of sexual attack.

Mothers are the resistance. Underground, invisible, forgotten. But I'd like to invite you to think, just for a moment, about where we'd be without them – those women who give life, rather than take it, who sustain themselves through everything to protect their children, whose primary function is to tend and befriend.

Even in relatively peaceful countries like my own, birth and motherhood don't always blossom organically. For some parents, being pulled in opposing directions, or lacking the kind of emotional support that bolsters their self-confidence, can result in a very wobbly start indeed.

Writer Susan Mildenhall says:

'Becoming a mother can change you so completely that your relationships can drift, shift or end in a rift, increasing your feelings of vulnerability and making it that much harder to deflect negative judgements or hostility directed your way.'

For some, nature deals them a rotten hand – full of complications, challenges, suffering and grief. Others have their births or babymoons effectively undermined or sabotaged, leaving the mother feeling traumatised. Trauma is a very personal thing, but for many it is the conflicting advice and medical interventions that they feel, or later find out, to be unnecessary that lead to mental suffering. Henci Goer, medical writer and researcher into maternity care, uses a common birth intervention as an example that sums up how inherently contradictory and confusing the world of obstetrics can be:

'In a branch of medicine rife with paradoxes, contradictions, inconsistencies, and illogic, episiotomy crowns them all. The major argument for episiotomy is that it protects the perineum from injury, a protection accomplished by slicing through perineal skin, connective tissue, and muscle.'

Everywhere I look, in my daily interactions with parents, I see people tugged in opposing directions; torn between what their guts and hearts are saying and the current prevailing cultural hegemony. Advice, from both medical professionals and friends and family, can be contradictory and based on an underlying assumption that birth is dangerous. We are told pregnancy is an illness from which hospital must rescue us. Then, when we dutifully present ourselves in labour, too many of us are turned away or admitted and ignored, due to staffing shortages and other pressures on the service.

'My instincts... pulled at me so hard and I resisted them equally as hard because they were "wrong". Things like co-sleeping, wanting to hold my baby, having the desire to breastfeed still at eight months despite stopping at four weeks... I remember feeling so abnormal for having these feelings that went so against what society says is right.' Claire Alexander

Blaming mothers and midwives and their desire for 'natural birth' for tragedies and mistakes is a serious injustice. Birthing people who choose medical birth also experience malpractice. Sometimes, medical interventions lead to a cascade of other risks that need to be handled with more interventions. Sometimes, even with the most skilled medical supervision in the world, things can go wrong. When mothers are coerced and emotionally manipulated into making decisions, the outcomes should never, ever, be blamed on the pregnant person.

I work in this landscape of contradiction and confusion daily. All too often I walk into houses where the anxiety is palpable. A veritable barrage of information is hampering women from 'melting into motherhood'.* Mother Clare Wells looks back and realises now that the instant love that people talk about isn't how it works for everyone: '...*loving my newborn baby was not instant. I felt fiercely protective of her and would have done anything to keep her safe, but the love grew.*'

Sometimes this is because a woman is coming back down from a dramatic or traumatic birth. Sometimes the domestic or social situation the baby is born into makes it difficult for one or both of the parents to bond. Sometimes, after difficult childhoods themselves, parents have no template for parenting, or a template that is shaky and shadowy. That pesky hormone of love is irritatingly shy and can be scared off by high stress. While that may seem a rather cruel trick for Mother Nature to play, oxytocin can be encouraged to flow through close contact, touch – especially skin-to-skin – breastfeeding, eye contact and the day-to-day interactions that a baby demands. And thus, the love grows. I don't think it's bad, or abnormal, not to instantly love our babies. I didn't love my husband at first sight either.

---

* Melting in motherhood is a term coined by the authors of the La Leche League book, *Sweet Sleep*, published by Pinter & Martin.

So often, it seems, notions of 'good' parenting are polarised: gurus and experts with dubious credentials, professionals, friends and family may all have strong convictions about how and what we 'should' be doing. From pregnancy health to birth, to vaccinations, to which school to enrol the kids in: everyone seems to have an opinion. As doula and breastfeeding counsellor Nikki Mather puts it:

'Why is the baby sleeping with you? Why aren't they in their cot/chair/Moses basket? You will make a rod for your own back. Your baby will never settle by themselves... A mum recently asked "How do I get my baby to sleep alone?". She was two weeks old. [We are] under pressure to carry babies without a hitch, birth like a pro and mother like the baby doesn't exist.'

Increasingly, women are waiting to have their children, and while I personally vehemently support a woman's right to choose when and how to have her kids, there may well be particular challenges for women who choose to be, or end up as, older mothers.

Janine Ebling told me that, in her experience:

'career women who have babies later in life, used to being so very in control of everything... it all goes belly up when a baby comes along and turns life upside down... These women often work... away from local community and have very few local friends to support them practically or emotionally in the early weeks.'

These days grandparents are often far away geographically or families are emotionally fractured. Sometimes this is the second generation of late motherhood and grandparents are too old and infirm to be of practical help. Or sometimes the opposite is true, but they still work full time and are therefore unavailable to their daughters or daughters-in-law.

Many of the women I support live in 'commuter land'; vast estates built on the outskirts of towns and cities, often lacking basic amenities. Even a quick trip to the shops involves strapping the baby into the car seat. There are few local support groups or cafes where parents hang out. The environment can be quite sterile in new communities: just as the trees around the estate are still saplings, the communities they have been planted in are still in their infancy.

Behind the curtains in these endlessly identical starter homes many women are finding it tough, thinking they are alone and desperately covering over the cracks with painted-on smiles. One mum, Ellie Cook, told me

> *'the postnatal experience is so secret. And I'm not talking about privacy. I'm talking about women feeling like they are supposed to "cope". They need people to think "she's got this, she's a pro, she's bounced back, she's back to normal." I wish everyone knew how open and wobbly we are... I wish it was common knowledge that one comment on the colour of your child's babygro can send you into floods of tears. I wish we were allowed to admit that we might not be enjoying it in the way we thought we would. Then others wouldn't feel the same sense of guardedness when their time came.'*

And, as breastfeeding counsellor Justine Fieth observes, women have:

> *'an overwhelming conviction that they must be doing it wrong...We have eroded mothers' instinct and confidence to the point that mothers feel lost...waiting for someone to fix or solve normal maternal and infant behaviour when they are the answer to their own question... as a society we have kicked mothers until they are down and then stand and judge them.'*

It seems we are expected to join a team, with proponents eulogising over parenting styles or choices with religious zeal. SAHM? AP? FF? EBF? BLW? Know what any of them mean? If you do, you've probably witnessed the evangelical fervour with which some people can talk about these subjects. As a result, hackles are raised, tempers lost, barriers created, everyone feels judged and often, commercial businesses are the only winners.

Doulas often see behind the veil to the reality of what it feels like to be a mother suffering social isolation and lack of family support, trying to grow her mother-wings in a cultural context that is profoundly anti-motherbaby. Doula Samantha Gadsden told me about a mother who had

'terrible PND... she hadn't coped... I was telling her that she needed to rest, recuperate, let everyone help her. She explained that last time people were shouting at her to get up and not understanding why she just wanted to stay in bed and feed her baby for two weeks. She was recovering from a caesarean section. BED and feeding her baby is exactly where she needed to be, most of the time.'

In this context of limited social support from family, friends and neighbours, the pressure falls squarely on the shoulders of the professionals – mostly midwives and health visitors. As the Royal College of Midwives explain on their website:

'Being a midwife is more than just delivering babies. A midwife is usually the first and main contact for the woman during her pregnancy, throughout labour and the early postnatal period. She is responsible for providing care and supporting women to make informed choices about their care.'

That's a big ask when the birth rate in the UK has been consistently climbing since 2000 and the number of midwives and health visitors has been falling. Maternity services have been the Cinderella service in the NHS for more than a generation. In particular, postnatal services have been woefully underfunded and understaffed. Currently the whole service is being held together with sweat, tears, unpaid overtime and sticky tape. The commitment of these midwives goes above and beyond the call of duty, and there aren't many people who really understand the pressures they are under. Asking them to provide psycho-social support on top of everything else can be the straw that breaks the camel's back. If there is one reason doulas and midwives should be natural allies, it's because we see midwifery at the sharp end and witness first-hand the many ways the system can chew up and spit out wonderful practitioners.

In this landscape, it's hardly surprising that some professionals find it hard to stay up to date. They certainly often lack the time to really sit and listen to women. Sometimes they may suffer from training that is outmoded, or let tiredness, being in a rush, or pressure from above to follow draconian guidelines obstruct them from putting the service users at the centre of all they do. Sometimes they are carrying the burden of personal trauma or memories of grief and violence they may have witnessed.

It might seem overblown and out of all proportion that so many midwives, doulas and mothers campaign for birthrights so vociferously: but we see so clearly that when a baby is born, so is a mother. How she feels, physically and emotionally, about the way her child comes into the world, has a profound effect on her for the rest of her life. It colours her sense of self and self-esteem, her relationship with her child, her partner and the world around her. It will inform the way she parents and thus have a deep and abiding effect on the person that baby will become and therefore the relationships that child will develop in adult life. Thus birth creates ripples that cascade down the generations.

The way we are born and the way we are fed as babies has an almost miraculous ability to even out social inequalities. This stuff matters. When the infant mortality rate for Pakistani, Black Caribbean and Black African babies in the UK in 2013 was almost twice the average,[8] we can be pretty sure we need to look very hard at the way our maternity services are working. When babies born into the least affluent families are the least likely to be breastfed, and when their mothers are the least likely to engage with health services, we know we have a problem. Providing skilled help for mothers to reach their breastfeeding goals does more to smooth out economic inequalities for that baby than any other single public health intervention, so we need to ask why it is not a social, political or health service priority.

The hoops and hurdles around childbirth worldwide are diverse. Agencies such as the World Health Organization and Maternity Action describe various challenges around childbirth, in particular the 'Three Delays',[9] which often cause trauma and tragedy. These delays are:

1. A delay in the decision to seek out care
This may be due to the low status of women or a poor understanding of the possible complications and risk factors in pregnancy and therefore when to seek medical help. It might be because a woman has had a previous poor experience of health care and is frightened to engage with doctors and midwives again this time. Or a pregnant person may not have had an opportunity to develop a trusting, compassionate relationship with a primary caregiver in this pregnancy and therefore does not feel able to reach out. There might be financial implications that restrict access to professional care. And sometimes, in some cultural contexts, there is an

acceptance of maternal death – that it is a reality of life that cannot be changed.

2. *A delay in reaching care*
This might be because of the distance to health centres and hospitals, or the availability and cost of transportation. It may be due to poor roads and infrastructure or the geography of the area.

3. *A delay in receiving adequate health care*
Perhaps because of inadequate facilities and lack of medical supplies, or maybe inadequately trained and poorly motivated medical staff. Sometimes there are inadequate or inappropriate referral systems.[10]

What the 'Three Delays' model beautifully illustrates is that just providing health care without empowering communities to access it can only increase health inequalities. While we might assume that these delays are solely a problem for developing countries, many of them happen regularly in richer nations too. Poverty, scant resources and under-developed infrastructure, wherever it is, always manifests in a similar way: restricting choices and obstructing people from accessing basic care.

Sometimes it feels, to any doula working in Europe or the United States, that the women we serve leave their homes and enter hospital like lambs to the slaughter; slavishly following the sheep, ignorant of what awaits them. The system, when functioning at its worst, can be toxic in a way that almost defies description and analysis. It is a poison that is more deep-rooted and systemic than poor care from individuals. It cannot even be blamed on management. It is a societal blindness to the very basic ingredients necessary to ensure safe, respectful, compassionate care. The poison runs in rivulets; over-intervention with medical technology, while sometimes saving lives, leaves a legacy of unnecessary morbidity and psychological damage to mothers, fathers and babies. In developing countries, either the life-saving care isn't there at all, or the worst excesses of Western obstetric medicine are applied without thought, cultural appropriateness or the necessary compassion, leaving death and destruction in their wake.

According to the World Health Organization, every day approximately 800 women die of preventable causes related to pregnancy and childbirth. Amnesty International's report, *Deadly Delivery: The Maternal Health Care Crisis in the USA*, urges action to tackle a crisis that sees between two and three women die every day during pregnancy and childbirth in the USA. The White Ribbon Alliance, a charity working to ensure the rights of all women, worldwide, to a safe birth, considers the lack of respectful care in labour to be one of the most serious barriers to accessing health care in pregnancy.[11] With a lifetime risk of maternal death that is greater than 40 other countries, including virtually all industrialized nations, the USA has failed to reverse the two-decade upward trend in preventable maternal deaths, despite pledges to do so.

Unlike the US, Britain has an independent body that records all maternal and perinatal deaths so that clinicians can learn and be held accountable. The Centre for Maternal and Child Enquiries[12] is crucial because it is only by recording and enquiring into the true cause of every maternal and infant death that we can draw conclusions that may improve maternity services. But we only improve if we act on the lessons learned. In the UK, successive governments have admitted that the NHS is short of more than 3,000 midwives. Promises to recruit have been consistently forgotten. Experienced midwives are leaving and retiring at an alarming rate. Midwives and mothers are worried that maternity services are being pared down to dangerous levels. At the time of writing, the Nursing and Midwifery Council,[13] the official regulator, which exists to *'set standards of education, training, conduct and performance'* for nurses and midwives in the UK has just one midwife advisor and appears determined to undermine and restrict the traditional role of midwife. Meanwhile, in many developing countries, millions of pregnant women have no access to antenatal care or skilled intrapartum (labour and birth) support at all.

In many parts of the world, the most basic healthcare is not freely available to women. All the evidence seems to suggest that some simple antenatal care can make a massive difference to the outcomes of pregnancy. A good diet, an eye kept on blood pressure, urine and the growth and position of the baby, someone to gently connect to, to listen and educate mothers on birth and baby care. This is not expensive, complicated stuff. Yet in many countries it simply does not exist. Even in the richest countries there are gaping holes in this most basic of care.

When pregnancy is not planned or intended, access to services can be even more limited. In many countries around the world, women have to jump through hoops to access contraception and abortion or it is denied to them completely. In some cultures, including my own, pregnancy outside clearly defined social parameters is still taboo – and taboos lead to silence, and a lack of education and support, ironically often leading to the very outcome the taboo abhors. For example, despite teenage pregnancy being looked down upon and seen as a social problem by British people, we still have the highest teen pregnancy rate in Europe.[14]

Judgement, restriction of a woman's dominion over her own body, silence and lack of education clearly doesn't result in the desired outcomes. What happens, more often than we would like, is that young girls delay getting antenatal care or even conceal their pregnancies entirely.

In the US many women do not have a choice about how and where to give birth because the insurance system dictates what is available. In some states, there are no postnatal home visits, midwives do not routinely provide primary care and routine practices that are not evidence based and considered risky in other countries are common – for example, routine vaginal examinations in pregnancy and use of pitocin to induce or augment labour. Despite evidence to the contrary, vaginal birth after caesarean is not supported in many hospitals. Deciding how and where to have a baby seems to be rather a lottery in America, with a dizzying variety of attitudes to birth choice, depending on state. American doula Lauren Beth Ordeneaux told me: *'Some states have lots of birth centers and a supportive infrastructure for home birth, while others have effectively made it illegal.'*

US mothers are usually allowed just six weeks' maternity leave before they lose wages and job security. As US doula Katie Llewellyn Rachanow explains, *'Most women in the US do not get paid maternity leave. The six weeks is usually unpaid and is a law called the Family Medical Leave Act... employers just can't fire a new mom but they don't have to pay her.'*

This means that women are going back to the workplace still bleeding from childbirth, still recovering from major surgery or episiotomies, and are having their freedom and right to breastfeed curtailed. However, given that the US rates of breastfeeding are much better than the UK's, despite our relatively generous maternity leave provision, I say hats off to American women!

A mother in Israel told me that birth there is also very mechanised.

'newborns are admitted to a baby unit at birth, and mothers come to collect them for feedings... it is a struggle to be well informed and fight for your rights, standing up to an "antique" minded labour ward. ...if mum and baby are admitted to the general ward, [they are] encouraged to get rest while the staff take care of the baby... Home birth is very much reprimanded and the few doctors and midwives who support it are prosecuted...'

In the UK, lack of continuity of carer means that many women see a different midwife every time they have an antenatal appointment. Midwives are so busy and so pressurised that appointments typically last only ten minutes or so. This means that mothers may not feel able to discuss their worries or feel safe enough to disclose things like drug-taking or domestic abuse.

But at least we have midwives and basic antenatal care. In many countries, midwives are outlawed, witch-hunted or sidelined. The traditional understanding that psycho-social care in pregnancy leads to better outcomes is being forgotten. Independent Midwife Virginia Howes has written of her experiences supporting birth in Pakistan:

'Rumi has had four children, two of which she had at home and two in a village hospital. The two she had at home sound as if they were easy, straightforward and, most interestingly, the things she says and advice she gives to Sofia are spot on. Like walking and squatting cuts the pain and how hot water makes the milk flow from the breast and the baby flow from the body... However, as soon as she talks about her hospital births... her whole manner changes and instead she talks about what she was allowed to do... It upset me to hear that they make the women remove their clothes and they are kept naked from as soon as contractions start. They are given no

privacy from male hospital workers and if they refuse to do what they are told they are often slapped!'

Once the baby is born, the full force of corporate greed often rains down on the family. In the UK, the perspiration from childbirth may still be glistening on your forehead when the Bounty lady knocks on your door requesting your contact details and showering you in commercial advertising and free gifts. Despite the best efforts of the World Health Assembly to curb the unethical marketing practices of the formula manufacturers, in many countries you may still leave hospital with a bag full of formula samples. Much as that may seem kind and generous, research consistently finds that free gifts of formula contribute to low breastfeeding rates. In other words, they help to sabotage mothers' new and fragile breastfeeding relationship with their babies. If you've ever been awake at 3am worrying about your milk supply, or suffering with sore nipples, you'll know how that tin of baby milk in the cupboard beckons temptingly. And no, I am not saying a mother should never use artificial baby milk. I am saying that a readily accessible crutch can derail a mother's own desire to learn how to nurse, affect her milk supply and risk the health of the baby.[15]

The corrupt and overblown marketing techniques of the formula companies take away freedom of choice and steer mothers and their babies into danger. Here in the West, we luxuriate in the knowledge that most babies who do not have access to breastmilk will be OK. But in many developing countries, and everywhere in times of war or natural disaster, breastfeeding is quite literally the difference between life and death.

I think it's time we said it out loud: mothers have been marginalised – by society and by feminism – for too long. Motherhood is almost a dirty word in a gender-neutral age.

Yet here in the ghetto of motherhood, we are discriminated against, vulnerable and financially dependent. Everywhere you look, mothers earn less and do more. Yes, fathers have it tough too. There is another book to be written about them, and the challenges that face modern fatherhood. But we must be clear: the way mothers are treated in so many countries is shameful, sad and needs to change. No other such group could be so consistently ignored without a loud and organised campaign... but mothers are too damn busy to mobilise!

If intersectional feminism is what it says on the tin, it's time to include mothers too – every flavour and colour by the way, not just white mothers but black and Asian mothers, gay mothers, bi-mothers, gender-queer and trans mothers and fathers. Because feminism isn't about escaping biology. It's about individuals having equal access to health and social care and being truly free to make choices: whether that's having kids or not, pushing babies out of your vagina or not, breastfeeding or chestfeeding or not, going out to work or staying at home with small people. And it means society welcoming, celebrating and rewarding all these choices, as equal contributions to society.

Sarah Caldwell is a doula who believes that *'we are poisoning mothers' minds...'* I can see her point. Daily I encounter women who are apologising for existing; feeling disgusted by their own bodies, embarrassed by their own emotions and wracked with guilt at every action and decision.

I have one, single apple tree in my garden. She is solid and upright, in the prime of her life, and just beginning to bear good fruit. This year she was more laden than ever before, fecund and fertile. Her apples ripened and fell in huge numbers, before we could harvest them all. With more sweet fruit than we could deal with, our tree is pregnant with possibility; tall and straight, her boughs strong and reaching for the sunlight. This summer, I lay under her shade, with half-closed eyes, peering up through her canopy of leaves, dozing and thinking about what it means to become a mother and contemplating the things that can poison the experience.

Like the worms that eat the apples, the toxic chemicals we may spray on the fruit or environmental pollutants that may affect their quality, there are aspects of motherhood that can be poisoned. Some poisons come from outside us, while other toxic aspects come from within.

When they first become mothers, many modern women have never been close to a new baby in their lives. The fruit of their wombs is alien to them, the ways of the baby strange and foreign-feeling. The emotional and physical impact can be immense.

Justine felt that new motherhood was *'Overwhelming exhaustion! And a desire to swear at anyone without children who said they were tired.'* Ellie remembers *'not enjoying it. And feeling guilty about not enjoying it.'*

We are stepping into our roles as parents against a backdrop of commercial and governmental sabotage. High pressure marketing of expensive baby equipment, a systematic underfunding and dismantling of maternity services and the erosion of choice in childbirth have a profound impact on the families I serve. Despite the official line that choice and high-quality services are governmental priorities, the reality on the ground is quite different. For example, independent midwives are currently (2017) battling the latest round of the ongoing concerted effort to eradicate them entirely. To the uninitiated, it may look like an unimportant battle to save eighty-odd self-employed midwives. The reality is that, for a significant proportion of the birthing population, support from such a midwife can sometimes literally be life-saving and often crucial to the optimal physical and mental health outcomes of the whole family they care for. These midwives are guardians of skills rarely used in the NHS and provide a template for continuity of carer. Their ridiculously good statistical outcomes for safety and satisfaction speak for themselves. Service planners and NHS management would do well to take note.

Closures of Children's Centres and breastfeeding support services around the country are also putting untold pressure on families and staff. Without trusted sources of factual information, parents are even more prey to the cultural constructs, myths and misunderstandings that can make bringing up children even more challenging. For example, the tired old trope that it doesn't matter what you feed a baby is a stab in the heart to mothers who are struggling to breastfeed (if it doesn't matter, why do I feel so disappointed and sad? I must be mad!).

There are so many, but a random selection of messages that undermine easy, instinctive parenting include: 'bedsharing is dangerous', 'nursery prevents clinginess', 'only working mums contribute to society', 'Stay at home mums are a drain on society', 'single mums are benefit cheats', 'babies and children must sleep through the night', 'parenting and education is best done on a reward and punishment basis', 'homework improves educational outcomes', 'school uniform prepares children for the world' and 'attachment parenting is for hippies and spoils children'. None of these assumptions has one jot of evidence to back it up. It's like some kind of toxic Chinese whispers; an invisible yet tangible pressure to conform.

Is it any wonder that so many new parents suffer mental distress? According to the World Health Organization, around *'10% of pregnant women and 13% of women who have just given birth experience a mental disorder, primarily depression.'*[16] In developing countries this is even higher, with nearly 20% of mothers suffering depression after childbirth. Suicide is a leading cause of maternal death around the world.

With these hurdles to face and hoops to jump through it can take years to find our feet and gain confidence, not only in our parenting approach and the decisions we make along the way, but also to stop feeling guilty about the cards life has dealt us.

It has taken years for Anna Richardson, a mother of four from Cambridge, to learn *'that if you're a single parent, it's ok to struggle'.*

Doula and childbirth campaigner Paula Cleary believes that:

'Inadequate paternity leave means mums having to return too quickly to running a household, doing school runs etc… all of which make life stressful and disruptive to the early skin-to-skin dyad. The babymoon is also not honoured or valued because a schedule of silly NHS appointments keeps mums having to get dressed, take baby out in the car, risking infection with each new place and professional and waiting room they have to go to, when baby should be close to mama's naked chest in the first days and even weeks of motherhood. This all acts as massive disruption to breastfeeding and undermines it.'

Vicki Markham Williams is an International Board Certified Lactation Consultant (IBCLC) who often finds herself reassuring mothers who have been told to leave their babies to cry.

'When babies feed well from the start and are nicely glued to mummy they don't cry much. I want to say so many things (some very rude) to health professionals who say crying is normal and babies ought to do it and should be allowed to.

It makes no biological sense whatsoever. A crying primate is asking to get eaten, so if crying doesn't bring mum they have to shut down, keep safe and conserve energy. That's not soothing, it's surviving!'

In a culture that seems intent on separating mothers and babies, the logical end point is a separation of a mother from her instinct. Doula Nikki Mather has noticed that we appear to have forgotten how to listen to mothers: *'If mum says something isn't right, she means it. She isn't being dramatic. She isn't "doing it wrong".'*

Becky Talbot, ex-sex and relationship counsellor, working in a young parent project (funded by public health money) tells me how younger mothers are routinely encouraged to separate from their babies.

'I provided sex and relationship education to young parents who attended throughout their pregnancy and the first year of their child's life. The main emphasis was on either getting quickly back into education or finding work. Although parenting skills were encouraged, breastfeeding certainly wasn't. The women were taken on holiday for the weekend six weeks post-birth without their babies on condition they had given up breastfeeding. Those that hadn't, couldn't come.'

Of course, the irony of policies such as this is that a deep, secure attachment between mother and baby is protective against a number of vulnerabilities and negative consequences, especially in families that may be more chaotic and dysfunctional than average.

Every day and in every way, the status quo is shored up by myths that discourage parents from being close with their children. Activities that are normal for our species and were common just a few generations ago are now considered taboo.

My friend Marie de Jonge recounted the tale of being *'out at a meal the other night and my friend was talking about her friend who was going to breastfeed past a year, all the women at the table pulled a face of disgust.'*

Wherever they are in the world, mothers fight for their children, even killing themselves in the belief that their children will be better off without them. Suicide is a leading cause of maternal death in many countries. Are we too ashamed to air these herstories, too scared to examine what it reveals of a world that allows such tragedy?[17]

In developing countries, mothers die for lack of basic medical care. Severe postpartum bleeding and infections, eclampsia, obstructed labour and other birth complications and unsafe abortion are the leading causes of death: all easily preventable. Since 2000 maternal death has reduced by over 40%, which is really good news, but these statistics hide the sad fact that around 800 women are still dying every day from preventable, pregnancy-related problems. That's nearly 300,000 a year, worldwide.[18]

When a mother dies in the West, the most common effect on the rest of the family is grief and a psychological impact on the partner and children that may last a lifetime. In developing countries, the impact can be even more far-reaching. Research has shown that when a family loses the mother, financial suffering often ensues. This leads to children being taken out of school or being sent away to live with relatives. Daughters are often married off, thus perpetuating the spiral of poverty and the health impacts of pregnancy on young girls: women who begin having babies before the age of 15 have a much greater lifetime risk of death during childbirth than women who begin childbearing later in life.[19]

Vanessa Olorenshaw, author of *Liberating Motherhood, Birthing the Purplestockings Movement* has been so incensed by the way mothers are discriminated against that she started a whole movement. From a standing start, there is a wave growing in size and intensity as more and more mothers realise that these frustrations, discriminations and injustices are not just happening to them.

I wonder what would happen if our bodies were celebrated for the effortless way we can bear children and feed them, instead of our curves and breasts being used to sell products?

What if mothers had a voice? What if we all took back what is ours – our birthright – to labour and give birth safely with skilled, loving attendants, in the place of our choice, in the manner of our choice; to be supported with patience and loving care through the transition to parenthood; to be surrounded by compassionate, skilled breastfeeding help and peer support; to be supported with affordable childcare, equal pay, financial support to stay at home with the children if we choose to. To live without fear of starvation, rape, slavery, or domestic abuse?

What if mothers had the time and energy to actually get a say in the way the world was run? I wonder how the world would look if mothers were freed from being financially dependent, marginalised and discriminated against.

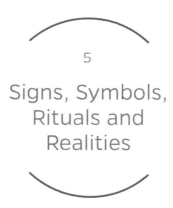

5

Signs, Symbols, Rituals and Realities

'A woman in harmony with her spirit is like a river flowing. She goes where she will without pretence and arrives at her destination prepared to be herself and only herself.'

Maya Angelou

Standing by the window in the delivery room, in labour with my first child, I looked out over the fields behind the hospital. Today the view is very different as the hospital site has grown, but in those days I could see trees and sky and the burst of yellow daffodils, nodding in the March breeze. I clutched the windowsill as another contraction flowed through me and suddenly, something very strange happened. I was simultaneously here, and not here. I was microcosm and macrocosm; vanishingly small and at once huge and at one with the universe. I was every mother who had ever birthed since the dawn of time and simultaneously every mother who ever would birth, on and on forever until the end of the world.

My out-of-body experience was not something I readily

shared with others, until I became a doula and heard other women talking about experiences that were equally ecstatic or had a sense of communion with the universe. I began to see birth as a spiritual rite of passage. A time for us to move beyond ourselves and our self-built identities; a time to meet our primal selves. We journey to a place above ego, beyond culturally-constructed ideas of who and what we should be and how we should behave; beyond even our deeply held beliefs about gender identity or sexuality. We meet ourselves in our raw, deconstructed state and see the 'essence of me'.

It is this power to reproduce and communicate with something above and beyond normal human experience that I am convinced has resulted in the feminine being both revered and feared throughout human history. Seeing the full, unhindered power of the birthing person results in either a worshipful awe or a fear and desire to silence and erase that power. Sadly, in modern times, the tendency is more to the latter.

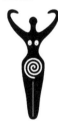

Once we were shamans, wisewomen, witches, priestesses. The role of the man in the creation of life was unknown or minimised. We fully inhabited our own sexuality, fecundity and fertility rites. We had our own rituals and ceremonies. Mothers were honoured and nurtured through the childbearing year. We had life-giving goddesses to mark our transitions and light our way through life.

Many of our most commonly used symbols have their roots in the divine feminine. Here is the circle, a primeval symbol of female power; unity, community and the feminine force innate in all women. Continue the circle and it becomes the sacred spiral, with its overtones of eternity, growth and evolution. Seeing women spiralling their hips instinctively to help their babies rotate and descend during labour always reminds me of its power and causes me to reflect on the myriad instances of spirals in nature from the unfurling fern to the spinning galaxies.

Three spirals become the Triskelion. The waxing, full, and waning moon. Birth, death and afterlife. The moon that, before electric light, had such a profound effect on our cycles and our birthing times. The moon was once 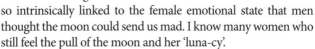 so intrinsically linked to the female emotional state that men thought the moon could send us mad. I know many women who still feel the pull of the moon and her 'luna-cy'.

 The spiral becomes ever more complex and morphs into the labyrinth; an ancient symbol of the female journey. It combines the imagery of the circle and the spiral into a meandering but purposeful path. It is not a maze; it does not need to be figured out. It has no dead ends or choices of paths to confuse us. Like birth, we walk the labyrinth one step at a time, one contraction at a time. We do not look behind us, nor do we look ahead. A labyrinth allows us to suspend all fear of the journey and learn to trust in the path we follow, albeit with a healthy respect for the hard work ahead! Liberated from having to puzzle out the path or fix a problem, the labyrinth allows us to sink into the daydream brainwaves of meditation; the instinctive knowing of the limbic system.

The journey of the labyrinth is a journey to our centre and back again; at times it feels as though we are travelling further away from our goal, moving out instead of towards the centre. There is undeniable, normal trepidation as we round each bend. But faith and trust in the path always leads to the centre, to transcendence, to birth, renewal, self-knowledge and insight.

At its centre we birth our babies, rest a while and then, when we are ready, we begin the journey back out, firstly carrying our babies, then walking at toddler pace, forced to view the world through the eyes of a child, carrying conkers and snail shells as tokens of the journey.

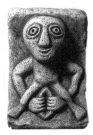

Unlike more stylised symbols, the Sheela-na-gig is in-your-face, proudly displaying her vulva, eyes wide, beatific smile on her face. Sheela of the 'gig', or vagina, guarded the entrance to churches in Ireland and other parts of the British Isles, but she is the sister of Kali, the Hindu divine mother, the destroyer, the 'one beyond time'. Sheela taught girls to celebrate their power and not to be afraid of their bodies. Sheela reminds us that, during childbirth, our vagina is perfectly designed to expand with ease to encompass the advancing baby's head. We can get so huge, in fact, that if men's sexual parts could increase in size so dramatically, they would boast about it! And just like a penis, the vagina can magically revert to its original size.

These symbolic figures, and many more, are the language of women. Secret, hidden and part of the celebrations and rituals with which we have always communicated, supported each other and passed on the wisdom to the next generation. For millennia, shamans, priestesses, healers, wise women and witches had a certain amount of autonomy and power over their own sexuality and fertility. Some opted out of the patriarchy by remaining celibate. Others were the sacred prostitutes of the temple, whose children bore their mother's name. Slowly, over the generations, these women were subjugated and silenced, their knowledge ignored and ridiculed. The monotheist mega-religions incorporated the female power-symbols, included women by giving them a secondary role and pacified the population by using watered-down versions of the ancient rituals and celebrations.

As I stood and laboured, rocked by intense waves of birthing power, I now realise I was Kali, 'she who is beyond time', both the creator and the destroyer. The fear of birth is something modern childbirth educators are trying to erase. I don't see this working: fear in the face of the terrible, beautiful, primal force of birth is something coded deep into our DNA. It is not just a primal terror of death, etched beneath our surface by our evolutionary epigenetics; it is a logical response to the awesome power and profoundly transformative nature of birth. Who could not tremble in its presence?

My role, as a doula, is to try to support women to respect that power, and to understand that while we may be subsumed by it for a while in the centre of the labyrinth, we return from our epic quest and come back to ourselves. This journey, which is simultaneously inward to our very core and outward, to the stars, is not something we can control, nor would we want to. It is a wild ride, and those who are present must venerate the process and sit at the feet of the birth goddess, in deference to her wishes.

Everywhere I look, however, I see people trying to control childbirth – and motherhood in general. There is an overwhelming desire to tame the tempestuous power, to gloss over the blood, the sweat, the tears and amniotic fluid and make the process sterile, planned, predictable. Over the centuries we have tried to explain and contain it, stripping it of its mystery and potential for profound insight. Birth, however it plays out for us, is an opportunity for epiphanies and profound personal growth. Yet it has been simultaneously minimised as a sacred life event, divested of the ancient rituals that comforted and educated women, and magnified, with the risk and the need for medical surveillance and intervention taking centre stage.

The raw-roar of birth needed to be silenced. It made men uncomfortable. It didn't fit in with the growing belief that women should be demure, prim and proper. Straight-laced isn't just a figure of speech; we were tied up tight in whalebones, hiding our pregnancies. When it was no longer possible to hide our burgeoning bellies, we were imprisoned in our own homes; confined until well after the baby was born. The ancient babymoon that honoured the mother, supporting her physical and psychological transition, became a means of control and a way to heap shame on women.

The natural functions of the female body were becoming toxic. It was the perfect way to control the fierce female: to imprison her in the domestic sphere, to shame her into hiding her body and the natural functions of that body and then, ultimately, to sell her the idea that she actually preferred the role of coy, modest domestic goddess. They controlled our bodies by teaching us to self-police; the idea of what constituted the body-beautiful changed constantly and still does. Women are expected to keep up, sculpting and remaking themselves for the male gaze.

I see the results of this systematic subjection of half the human race every single day in my work. Women are afraid of making a noise during childbirth. They are even more terrified of doing a poo as they push their babies out. They are ashamed of their lactating breasts; covering them and feeling mortified if they leak. At the extreme end of the scale, we are still fighting for the abolition of female genital mutilation – the ultimate example of control over a woman's sexuality and fertility. What better way to subjugate a woman than to take away her source of pleasure and power?

Confined to the domestic sphere, imprisoned within the nuclear family, women in the West were cut off from the traditional support of an extended family. With no sisters or aunts in the house, mothers began to talk over the garden fence, to gather in each other's kitchens, and at the school gates. The talk, the company and, in Britain, the never-ending tea, provided the social glue that held our communities together. Today, social media provides some of that glue – a chance to learn from each other in a supportive community. But we tend to congregate into groups of similar women online: same age, same interests, same politics. It's rare that women can learn from mother-figures and support daughter-figures; a mother with a baby rarely gets an insight into life as a mother of teens.

While it is fundamentally a Good Thing that some mothers have a choice to work or contribute to their communities outside the home, most mothers are still denied that choice. Either they cannot get a job, cannot afford the childcare that would enable them to get a job, or they would prefer to concentrate on the job of raising their children, but are driven by economic necessity to seek employment. Both men and women are trapped in gender roles that minimise the sum of human happiness.

'I think there is a hugely contradictory message... Be educated, work to contribute to society but you'd better be a perfect helicopter parent... I was driven to work as a mother for many years based on my own fear of financial insecurity... It was an extremely unhealthy struggle. Since stepping off the traditional treadmill, I feel fulfilled as never before... work can be fulfilling and meaningful and doesn't have to mean a compromise. Once you step outside the 'norm' there is huge freedom to design the life you want.' Verity Croft

Being economically available is not the only way to be useful to society. It seems we have forgotten that nurturing children is also of benefit to humankind. This work once had status and women were celebrated for their ability to grow, birth, feed and nurture new humans. When was it that these superpowers started being taken for granted? And when were other members of the extended family and community locked out and discouraged from taking an active role in raising the kids? That which confines women within the strict definition of 'mother' also restricts men, homeosexuals and transgender people, preventing creative, cooperative parenting and encouraging prejudice and judgement.

'Our society treats being a mother as a lowly task, one that isn't valued because it doesn't bring income and isn't seen as something that requires skills. Yet is it the most intensely demanding job ever.' Sophie Messager

It seems to me that the families I support are having to run faster and harder every day, just to stand still. Commuting fathers never see their babies, mothers work long hours to pay for expensive nurseries, and babies in nurseries from 7am to 7pm never see their parents. Nursery staff are underpaid and overworked, children are pushed to achieve and fill their time from sunrise to sunset with organised activities. I yearn for bored children running off to make a den, for mothers to lie on the grass watching the clouds, for dads to have a chance to experience the ordinary, everyday stuff – the school runs, the baby groups, the playground gossip. I celebrate when the house is a mess because I hope it means a mother who is doing something that makes her heart sing or just sprawling on the sofa with a child and a book.

Single mothers are under particular pressure; responsible as they are for the whole shebang. Women of Generation X and the Millennials have been told they can 'have it all', without anyone explaining what 'all' actually entails or listing the sacrifices we might have to make along the way. Being unable to follow our heart's work can be a frustrating part of motherhood:

'I have to work, but I do also enjoy work and I feel I should use my skills for the community. I do feel under pressure to do everything... I'm very glad that I live at a time where I am not overly stigmatised for being a working single mother. I wish I had more community support... I can get very anxious on short-term contracts worrying about money.

It's all very well being able to step off the beaten path. And give in to your passion if you don't have to pay all the bills! I do feel a bit resentful that sometimes it's implied you aren't brave or committed but actually, sometimes it's just not possible if you don't have a partner or a trust fund!' Selina Wallis

But being single can bring liberation, too:

'Now I am a single parent, I work as a doula just trying to be the best me I can be. Not somebody else's vision of what a 'good' mum/wife should be. Now I'm being me, my children are growing into themselves. They sleep in my bed if they want, we get takeaway a lot, we talk about poetry and we drink juice out of wine glasses on a Friday night.' Zoe Walsh

'I felt... an incredible debt of gratitude to the women before me who were pilloried, institutionalised and criminalised for being single parents, and for those who stood their ground.' Melanie English

And for those who are able, and choose, to stay at home, the pressures can be very real too:

'I left my academic career to be a stay-at-home mother because I was suicidal. My family are all high-powered career types who use nannies. In that environment I do feel like what I do is considered worthless... I get a lot of comments from my family about my being too involved in my children, "over breastfeeding" them, that they are "mummy's boys". My

full-time mothering isn't considered to be "healthy" by some.'
Elizabeth Staunton Acheson

Sometimes it can seem that our traditional support systems have abandoned us. Communities and families are fractured or separated by geography, we have often lost the rituals that bound us together with our neighbours and, for mothers, it can seem that even feminism can leave us on the periphery. Here, Sara Vale talks about her homeland of Portugal, where mothers are rising up and demanding longer maternity leaves.

'More and more women make the choice to leave work altogether, brave the lower income in the household and stay with the kids. There was a big petition to increase the maternity leave but it is still in discussion. Strangely, hard-core feminist groups were strongly against it, saying it would be going back to the 50s... A world of contradictions...'

What I see most in the women around me is strength in the face of adversity and a stubborn refusal to accept the status quo. As my friend Millicent says, just keeping your head above water: *'takes commitment, adaptability, patience, creativity, financial wizardry and a whole lot of sheer bloody mindedness!'* Yet I am acutely aware that not all women have the ability to raise themselves out of poverty, discrimination or violent relationships. I think we need to be very conscious not to fall into the trap of believing there are those who deserve support and those who don't.

The choices we have now are luxurious compared to our mothers and grandmothers. We owe a huge debt of gratitude to those women who suffered and died to give us freedoms and equalities that they could never have dreamed of. Yet the fight for support from society at large is ongoing:

'On a day where my request to work part time has been denied and my employer is bullying (and denying it)... I'm going solo!'
Charlotte Ashley-Roberts

If we were to raise parents out of poverty we could create real choice. A choice to educate and nurture their children, a choice to volunteer in their communities, a choice to work, or create their own businesses, tell their own stories and share the tales of their mothers and grandmothers. A chance to express themselves in whatever way they chose. A choice to rediscover our old goddesses and to welcome them back into our homes and hearts. And I bet you a million pounds the net contribution they made to society would far outweigh any initial investment.

'I really resent the real and perceived expectations from society that we should all be working in paid employment in order to justify our existence. Looking after my children is very valuable work and those who choose to do so should not be made to feel second-class citizens.' Karen Law

It feels like the round, beautifully creative, capable peg of motherhood is being forced into the square hole of societal expectation and the capitalist machine. It seems such a waste of human potential.

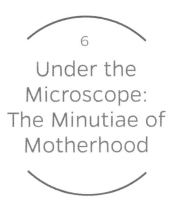

6

Under the Microscope: The Minutiae of Motherhood

'Not all of us can do great things. But we can do small things with great love.'

Mother Teresa*

Our work as mother-supporters, family-helpmates and 'guardian-angels', means that doulas and breastfeeding counsellors get to see family life under the microscope. We are privileged to see parents and children up close and personal, in the raw. I know that people, just like animals, may not act totally naturally when they are aware of being observed, but I think we get a pretty good insight into what life with a new baby really looks like. Over time, we begin to notice the minutiae of family interactions and begin to understand them as part of a bigger picture.

I notice how mothers communicate with their unborn child. They caress their bellies. Sometimes they prod gently and get an

---

* Apparently this isn't exactly what she said and is a paraphrased version that is commonly misattributed to Mother Teresa. I love it anyway.

answering kick. They shift an uncomfortable foot from under a rib. They can feel fingers tickling their bladder, a head nodding on a cervix, hiccups always at the same time of day, sleeping and waking patterns recognised and understood. I notice how, towards the end of pregnancy, a mother seems to know things, not visible to the naked eye. She might know when the baby is going to be born, or understand that, despite the calendar, her child needs just a little more time to cook. She might dream about her baby or about the birth and these dreams may give her surprisingly useful information. Her knowing is unquantifiable and intangible, but it is real and should not be ignored.

This conversation continues through the birth. I have noticed that pregnant people often seem to know that their babies are fine, even if the medical staff are concerned. Conversely they also seem to know if their baby needs help, even if those around them are convinced all is well. I have learned to lean in and listen intently when a labouring woman is telling me about her baby. She is the conduit; the way the child communicates with the world outside. I don't know how these messages reach her lips, but it seems logical to me – the child is part of her body. The myriad minute and subtle sensations and chemical signals that flow between parent and foetus must give her unconscious information that is at least as relevant as the medical observations.

It amazes me how often parents recognise the baby when they are born, like an old friend who has come to visit after a period of absence. I have witnessed more than one mother say to the baby, 'oh, it's *you*', just moments after the birth. And while the first day or two with a newborn can seem a whirlwind of anxiety and confusion, there is a deep and primal *knowing* that underscores everything.

'I love how quickly new mothers learn to know what their babies like and dislike. Within 24 hours, they say "he/she likes this/

doesn't like that". It often takes someone to point it out to them though, how quickly they have developed this skill.' Sophie, doula

Sitting with a mother with a new baby in her arms is yet another lesson in the micro-movements of their non-verbal conversations. The baby may look up at her, and her eyes are often inexorably drawn into the gaze-game. Baby may poke out a tongue or yawn or attempt a smile and she will inevitably mirror the facial expressions or comment on them. She might caress a hand and the baby will reach out and grasp her finger. To and fro they 'talk', with each trying to mimic the other's sounds and expressions.

Nikki, a doula, told me she loves watching the *'Synchronisation. Like a perfectly timed... performance being rehearsed for the first time. Slowly but surely coming together as one, as though they've been intertwined forever but are learning each other's ways once again.'*

Sarah Curtis loves watching *'The fresh faces wearing their father's noses. The personalities that surface. The cooing, the cuddling, the sing-song slow exaggerated face shapes that show babies "ooh" and "ahh" and to poke out their tongue.'*

Each time she looks away, the baby may attempt to regain her attention, yearning for her gaze, drinking it in, until, finally, exhausted, the baby turns away, sated, and seeks sleep or the comfort and warmth of her breast.

'Watching mothers – touching, stroking, sniffing, putting their faces together often without them being aware they are doing it. Newborn babies can look at their mother and communicate so much – and the mother instinctively responds... We need to protect that instinctive communication and interaction – they are a dyad. Even mothers struggling to bond will show that instinctive communication – and their realisation of that that can sometimes be at the heart of strengthening the bond.' Justine Fieth, La Leche League Leader

Sitting with parents and babies is like having a front row seat at the filming of a wildlife documentary. Like the private life of a butterfly or an iguana, the daily interactions between a new baby and the family are usually hidden and secret. The behaviours are complex, subtle and sophisticated. A mother soon learns to simultaneously watch the baby and carry on conversations with others. As my friend Linda says, even when she is talking to someone else, her eyes often never leave the baby.

If the mother/caregiver does not engage in this way, the effects on the baby are well-documented. The famous 'still face' experiment, in which the mother remains expressionless despite the child's best efforts to engage, results in high stress in the baby and, if taken to the extreme, affects cognitive development, most notably the empathy centres of the brain.[20] Research studies have found extremely high cortisol levels in the brains of babies who have been left to cry or ignored. These levels remain high, even after the 'stressing event' has ceased. This flooding of the baby with stress hormones affects both cognitive and physical growth. The extreme example of this are children raised in dysfunctional environments like the Romanian orphanages, whose brains were often severely damaged by the lack of loving interaction or exposure to the emotional regulation that results from a secure attachment to a parent-figure.

All parents spend the first days and weeks learning to 'speak baby'; understanding those cues – the little noises, facial expressions and body language that tell them what the baby is trying to say or what he or she is experiencing right now. Often by the time I have been supporting them for a few weeks, they can tell when the baby is tired, they know the 'poo face' and are anticipating the child's needs with ease. As I watch mothers in groups, at home or in the street, they are usually simultaneously interacting with the world and hyper-vigilant of the baby. A mother may be telling me about a breastfeeding issue while at the same time checking the child's nappy and calculating whether she has time to get to the shops before reaching the safety of her favourite nursing chair at home. It's why mums often have a far-away look in their eyes and why they are hard on themselves for forgetting things. But most of the time, they keep all the plates spinning with ease.

I am constantly reminded that this parenting lark often looks like nothing. It isn't big and brash with any obvious, loud evidence of achievement at the end of each day. As the renowned Naomi Stadlen says in her book, *What Mothers Do, Especially When it Looks Like Nothing*:

'A person who has "tidied up" has both the words and a tidy area to show for it. It is much harder to find a word that describes the giving-up-things mode of attention a mother is giving to her baby.'

I never see mothers being congratulated for simultaneously having a conversation about hopscotch with a five-year-old while paying for the shopping, wiping spit-up off a baby and putting the bags in the trolley. No one stops her and gives her a prize for what is happening in her head – always three steps ahead of the game, planning the evening meal, making a mental note not to forget to sign that permission slip for school, working out how many nappies she has left in order to decide whether to go back into the shop or go home and wait until tomorrow. Not many people celebrate when a mother in south Sudan manages to send her children to school in pristine school uniforms or a mother in India works hard to afford sanitary towels so her daughters can go to school.

No one jumps for joy at the arithmetical skill with which she works out if she has enough money left over for a treat. And does anyone care that she is bone deep tired, lonely and aching for adult conversation? Who celebrates with her when it's been a good day and she's enjoying the little people and who commiserates when the only solution feels like the comfort of a large glass of wine?

Who remembers the mother whose boys go off to war? Or those who have lost their babies and who carry the heavy burden of grief with them everywhere they go? Who remembers those who are struggling with other practical, financial, physical or emotional challenges?

Why is it that finger painting, bottom wiping and pulling the petals off daisies is considered less important than the chief executive of a company chairing a board meeting? When I was an English teacher a common classroom activity to stimulate discussion was the 'balloon debate': the balloon is losing altitude and we need to throw one person out of the basket to save the lives of everyone else. For many women, it feels like 'stay at home mum' has been grabbed by the ankles and unceremoniously thrown overboard.*

At our weekly support group we sit with mothers who come to us seeking breastfeeding help. All their instinctive knowing, faith in their parenting skills and ability to breastfeed may have abandoned them. They often arrive traumatised and feeling alone and betrayed by a system that they expected to support them to feed their babies. Sometimes, all they need is a listening ear and a kind, gentle word of validation. Rachel O'Leary, IBCLC, describes a magical moment she often sees:

'I love it when their bodies take over – for example trying and trying to get a baby latched on, then somebody suggests a break with baby on mother's chest – talk about something else, perhaps the birth experience – and suddenly the baby makes her way to the breast and latches on. The expression of

---

* Yes, I know. Loads of mums are utterly happy and fulfilled and won't recognise this description. And yes, dads, partners and LGBTQI parents have it super-tough too.

delight on the mother's face when she realises her baby is her teammate, working hard and skilful too.'

There probably isn't much more of a high for a new mum with sore nipples than when everything suddenly falls into place. Kathryn, a breastfeeding counsellor, revels in that look on a mother's face when she realises she no longer has to *'hate every second of it any more.'*

Of course, mothering manifests in many different ways. The special relationship between a surrogate and the parents is one example that is often profound and beautifully altruistic. These stories remind us that a birthing person is not always the mother of the child and impress on us what immense gifts women can bestow on each other. Zoe Walsh tells her story of surrogacy:

'The emotional investment in picking out which couple I would choose to journey with was one of the biggest hurdles I've faced. Every person looking for a surrogate had such a history, walked such a difficult path and their stories were overloaded with grief, loss, heartache and pain. So many babies miscarried, so many women with cancer and treatments which had left them unable to get pregnant or carry a baby. Nobody, I realised, came to look for a stranger to carry, grow and birth their child easily or without first experiencing difficulty and facing hard decisions.

The journey we took together, the intended parents, my children and I was sometimes fraught, often emotional and ultimately fulfilling... While I was sure they wouldn't leave me with a baby I didn't want, what if...? What if a complication arose which led to a caesarean or a long-term health problem, how would I feel then?

My children just boasted about what I was doing, while I plodded on and smiled to the outside world. I prepared myself for the hormonal and emotional shift after birth. My own children were the post-birth cuddles and love my body craved and I had the placenta encapsulated to further prop me up. My doula and my mum ensured I rested, went slowly and was nourished. I harvested colostrum antenatally and expressed breastmilk after the birth: some went home with the baby when she was born and the rest went to my local milk bank. This, I hoped, would also allow me to gently control the changes in my body, to allow me to physically adjust to the lack of a baby. While I knew in my head the baby was not mine, I wanted to allow my body time to get used to that idea too.

The labour and birth in my home, with my children, my doula, my mum, my midwife and the baby's mother was an unforgettable and invaluable piece of my life. Birthing a baby and handing her over to her mother, watching as she was held tightly and her mother fell in love was a great gift for me. I did what I needed to do and it was amazing.'

These precious shared moments with mothers teach us something profound. The relationship between a mother and child is important. The relationship between a baby and its father or other significant caregivers is important too. The relationships between mothers and parents of all kinds are also important. The bond between child and parent is an attachment that is primal, ancient and fathoms deep. When it works as evolution has designed it, it protects a baby from harm and facilitates optimal physical and cognitive development. It is a relationship that deserves to be protected; conserved, like a delicate and rare wild flower.

Because, like any extinction, losing the exquisite role of the mother could have ripple effects on the whole eco-system.

There are few more profoundly complex examples of those potential ripple effects than the breastfeeding relationship. Various threads in European culture over the last 50 years or so have conspired to deconstruct the mother-child nursing relationship and replace it with something anyone can do. Partly this came from a laudable feminist idea that women should not be forcibly tied to the domestic sphere against their will. The Victorian stereotype of the 'angel of the hearth' was rebelled against; why should a mother be tied to her child by seemingly never-ending round-the-clock feeds? Shouldn't the man step up and take his share?

The nursing relationship was further undermined by a glut of cows' milk that needed to be used and a growing trend for seeing birth and parenting as potential business opportunities. The ancient skills and knowledge of breastfeeding, once passed down through the generations, were being lost. Breastfeeding has become the meadowland of Special Scientific Interest, covered in rare wild flowers, which has been bulldozed and built on by cowboy builders. Without doubt, there are some who need those houses, but there should be room for the wild flowers too. The problem with allowing developers free rein is that, in their pursuit of profit, they will do everything they can to make people forget the need for meadows. In fact, they will do all they can to make us believe meadows are pointless, that green campaigners are eco-warrior nut jobs and that those who enjoy wild flowers are judging those who want houses. Unfettered promotion of formula, bottles and teats all contributes to the threatened extinction of some rare and beautiful flora and fauna – breastfeeding – and it appears no one is very interested.

The problem is, that not breastfeeding is not a liberation. At least, it isn't always as simple as that. If it were, breastfeeding support groups would be empty. We can present formula as a route to freedom and an equal choice, but the majority of mothers *want* to breastfeed, for all sorts of reasons: consciously, because of the undeniable and irrefutable evidence of the risks of formula feeding, and unconsciously, because, well, it just *feels* right. Research shows that mothers tend to choose to breastfeed not because of a rational weighing of the advantages and benefits, but with a deeper, more primal part of themselves. Putting our babies to the breast is, for most women, a biological urge as deep and primal as the desire to conceive in the first place. Social and cultural stories and pressures can undermine or even obliterate that desire, but to deny its existence is more than a shame – it is an insult.

Breastfeeding has become invisible and therefore easily forgotten. Worse, it has become a taboo subject. The marketing men have realised that if they imbue the subject with judgement and conflict, people won't talk about it. While campaigning for better local breastfeeding support services I recently heard a local councillor refer to breastfeeding as a subject 'where angels fear to tread'.

In a marketing masterstroke, the formula manufacturers have made nursing a baby something dirty; something to provoke shame and trepidation, something that provokes controversy and conflict. In all this, we have forgotten the very real economic value of breastmilk.

Vicki Markham Williams told me what she has found to undermine the desire and the ability of mothers to reach their breastfeeding goals.

> *'What do we get most wrong for breastfeeding? Birth. Then the promotion, then the support... Too few people know how to tell if a baby is effectively latched and feeding well, and even fewer really know what to do if they aren't... That leads to a giant cultural myth that breastfeeding is hard, painful and frequently doesn't work, and that message is pervasive and the spiral continues...'*

I wonder what would happen if we counted the myriad tiny and not-so-tiny daily tasks of mothering in the GDP of our countries? What if we added up all those hundreds of thousands of litres of breastmilk and calculated what that adds to the economy? In Australia, researcher Dr Julie Smith has estimated that up to $120m could be saved annually across the hospital system if all babies were breastfed until six months of age. A study in the *British Medical Journal* (*BMJ*) in 2014 estimated that:

> *'Supporting mothers who are exclusively breastfeeding at 1 week to continue breastfeeding until 4 months can be expected to reduce the incidence of three childhood infectious diseases and save at least £11 million annually.'* [21]

Liberating women from the ties of breastfeeding and the discourse on bodily autonomy has confused our attitudes towards feeding our babies. Breastfeeding has been rewrapped and sold back to us as a 'lifestyle choice'; something women do for their own pleasure and fulfilment. How might we change the paradigm if nursing mothers began to be seen as undertaking a task that contributes to society? What if, instead of minimising or undermining this activity, we started saying thank you? The ability to provide this free, endless, life and health-giving substance is the ultimate example of a mother's altruism; not just benefiting her child but, in measurable and verifiable ways, positively impacting on her own health and the state of society as a whole.

When we hide the tasks of mothering away behind closed doors they don't just become invisible, they begin to be perceived as unimportant. The subject of lactation – the means by which we have kept our babies alive since, well, forever – has all but fallen out of the curriculum of obstetric doctors. In 1995 a study[22] found that fewer than 40% of doctors were provided with any lactation management training, instead picking up information from midwives and other maternity staff. Doctors were significantly more likely to rate themselves as effective in providing breastfeeding support if they had nursed their own children. A more recent review[23] concluded that there is *a critical need for research to address breastfeeding education and training needs of multidisciplinary healthcare staff*'.

Yes, you read that right: doctors get next to no training and rely on colleagues and their own experiences. Doesn't sound so bad? If you had asthma, would you like to be cared for by someone who had once had an asthma attack or who had talked to an asthma nurse at a dinner party? And what if that asthma nurse was relying on hearsay, myth, tradition and old wives' tales, instead of clinical practice and evidence?

Women receive strong public health messages about breastfeeding during pregnancy. All the leaflets and parenting books outline the health benefits to the baby. They internalise a message that breastfeeding your baby is part of the identity of a 'good mother'. Yet the moment the baby is born, it appears to many parents that the health service does an abrupt U-turn and withdraws all support. Parents are ignored or undermined in a million different ways: doubt as to milk supply, lack of solutions for sore nipples, blame put on the mother for being too ginger, too lazy or too weirdly shaped, or not eating and drinking enough. And formula is pushed as the solution, the norm against which all else is measured. It is hardly surprising that fury, guilt, sadness and regret are the result when things don't go to plan. We blame ourselves, not even realising we are victims. Not even realising that the odds were stacked against us from the start. Breastfeeding is a skill humans learn by imitation, like walking and talking. But how can we imitate something we have never seen? How can doctors and midwives help us, when all they ever see is breastfeeding failing? And how can our babies teach us, with their strong, sensitive neonatal reflexes, when they are so often born before their time, drugged and sleepy?

In many countries, mothers go home with free samples of formula milk. By the time they have run out of the free white powder, they are hooked and their own milk supply is compromised. Purveyors of other white powders use the very same marketing techniques to increase their market share of addicted consumers.

We have got to a point as a culture where we understand the intense mental distress that infertility causes women and have invested in treatments. Yet breastfeeding problems and the lifelong emotional trauma associated with difficulties and 'failure' are ignored and dismissed. When poor, illiterate mothers walk past billboards featuring aspirational images of white babies thriving on formula, when formula tins are reassuringly expensive, and when the instructions for making up that powder are confusing or in a different language, free market capitalism becomes an agent of death. Poverty or unreliable supplies of formula lead mothers to water down the powder to eke it out.

In refugee camps in northern France, volunteer midwives appear blind to the additional dangers that haunt babies and young children living in shacks in a muddy field with no electricity or easily accessible running water. Formula has become such a taken-for-granted product, such a part of our daily lives, that it seems impossible to believe it could harbour bugs strong enough to kill a newborn baby.

Even in the cold, the damp and without basic facilities, mothers commune with their babies in the most beautiful way. They unwrap them tenderly, like a precious vase deserving of a place in the Louvre. They stare and touch a cheek or play with tiny fingers. But the shadows of war, terror, rape and near-death experiences flicker in the eyes of the mothers, weighed down by memories of terrible horror and deep, bone-crushing exhaustion. They look like they haven't slept for years. And even now, in the relative safety of Europe, volunteers bring them adult nappies because going to the toilet block at night is too dangerous. As Paula Gallardo, founder of the Refugee Community Kitchen, tells me:

'What I see everyday is women creating nations with their hearts and arms for their children and with gentle and grateful smiles. But behind those smiles we see weariness, we see how they miss the support from the ground of their homelands. I see the yearning for the arms of their grandmothers, their mothers, their sisters and the graves of their ancestors.'

Linda Robinson MBE has volunteered in both the Calais Jungle and the camp in Grande Synthe, Dunkirk. She told me that she

'saw mothers with their children in pushchairs wandering aimlessly around the camp. They spoke of the horrendous journey to flee from their country where they witnessed their homeland being destroyed and family members killed in front of them.'

Whether our lives are small and mundane, or we are buffeted by the storms of war or privation, it really is the little things that count. The banana a refugee mother gave me when I visited her shelter, the getting out of bed despite pain or crippling postnatal depression, the small smile of understanding when another mum's toddler has a meltdown in the supermarket, the kind word on social media, the food left on the doorstep when the whole family has flu (I'll never forget that, Candie!), the friend who looks you in the eye and says, 'how are you, *really*?' The minutiae of motherhood.

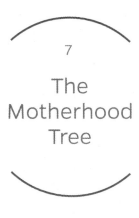

7

The Motherhood Tree

'Every thought is a seed. If you plant crab apples, don't count on harvesting Golden Delicious.'

Bill Meyer

The shifting sands of parenthood dicate that, while the majority of us will become parents at some point in our lives, the way that experience affects us will vary incredibly from person to person. However much we would like to steer away from difficult reflections on gender roles, it is unfair to talk in generalised terms about 'parenting' without unpicking it all a little more and teasing out the particular issues that affect mothers, fathers, same-sex and trans parents. But in the laudable drive for equality and lack of discrimination, let's not forget the individual challenges that face women-as-mothers-and-carers.

I sometimes use the analogy of the chrysalis to describe the process of transition that women go through during this time. During the early weeks of mothering, we are mostly hidden from the world, learning, growing, changing; trying on the role of parent for size. At some point, we break out and fly: capable and beautiful, revelling in motherhood. Of course, I realise this is an idealistic image, that ignores those who suffer inside their chrysalis or whose wings are different to others and feel the pain and sense of marginalisation of that. I realise not everyone learns to fly quite so easily. And most of us need help, at first or for always.

Ellen Thornhill told me:

'I'm trying to drop the notion that life will "get back to how it was" with just a baby added. Life is fundamentally different, and I think that's how it should be… I couldn't imagine how though and I think I'm still grieving a little for the old life I now realize is gone forever. I think there is a 'hushedness' around how hard it is, and how much of a full-on adjustment it can be.'

What is pretty similar for everyone, whoever we are and wherever we are in the world, is that the societies we fly out into are not set up to support and nurture mothers. In fact, it is the women who are pretty much doing all the work of caring for others, rather than receiving it themselves, be it for children or the sick, old and dying – and that work is pretty much denigrated, ignored and seen as degrading.

Dr Gail Ewing is a senior researcher at the Centre for Family Research, University of Cambridge. She says:

'Historically, care has been something that families undertake and, when it's good and families are well supported, nothing can substitute this kind of care. It's always been the case that most carers – both unpaid and paid – are women. When larger numbers of women spent their lives at home rather than the workplace, care was something they built into their other activities. But families have changed: most women have

jobs as well as family responsibilities and they find themselves juggling their roles. Despite these changes, women undertake the overwhelming responsibility of care. And it's women who more often than men find themselves alone and needing care at the end of life.'

I now think of our 'family tree' of mothers, stretching back into the mists of time. Each new mother starts out as a bud, then becomes a blossom and then a fully-grown apple, blushing pink, full and juicy.

There is no 'one-size fits all' approach to this crazy adventure that is motherhood; all our talents, hang-ups and phobias come along for the ride. I remember being distinctly aware in the early days after the birth of my first baby that the only template for mothering a newborn I had was how I, myself, had been mothered. I had nowhere else to turn for mothering to be modelled to me. For many of us, the apple doesn't fall very far from the tree.

The social isolation that comes from childcare being restricted to the domestic sphere means that we spend less and less time just 'hanging out' with other new parents. Out in the world we are admonished for not keeping our kids under control, tutted at if they are too noisy and judged for our tits or bottles. If we have added challenges, like physical disability or mental health issues, for example, the isolation can be unbearable. If we are judged 'too young' or 'too old' or experience racial or other types of discrimination, parenting a small child can feel very tough indeed.

'being quite a young mum I did experience a lot of judging in how I brought up my son. I was adamant that I wanted to breastfeed from the start. It was a hard start and formula was forced on me in the first few days by health professionals rather than just helping [me] learn to breastfeed. But I persisted until

I got it right. Black women breastfeed at a lower rate than white women do... I was pressured a lot to stop just because he could walk or because he had teeth now. Some of my family looked disgusted by it but I just ignored their ignorance because I knew what was right for me and my son... I was the only one of all my friends to breastfeed past one month and the only one to babywear so people were confused. There is a lot of stigma on young mums. People expect us to be standing on the corner of the street smoking weed and talking about the time we were on Jeremy Kyle or something. But not all mums are like that, most young mums just want to do their best but don't have the right support, guidance or just a simple friend to talk to.' Sasha Senior

There is a real lack of research and resources being put into exploring the particular needs of parents who suffer discrimination. Assumptions are too often made by health professionals that women of colour will not want to breastfeed.[24] These parents may not feel as welcome in baby groups or as able to access support services. Young parents are routinely assumed to be incapable or feckless and disabled mothers are patronised on one hand and abandoned on the other. Some parents are weighed down by layers of discrimination and can feel completely invisible and forgotten.

Aside from baby groups and NCT reunions, the era of communal living and mutual support appears to be over, especially once the baby months are over and many women are at work all day. Without our sisters to turn to, we work two jobs and collapse into bed without respite, rest or relaxation. And what keeps us at this relentless grindstone? The toxic mixture of money and guilt, sprayed on the tree to keep the apple growing. It's a pretty bitter apple that often results.

For some of us, the memories of our own childhoods will

give us useful guidance and strong opinions on how we want to parent. The 'I'm not doing it *that* way' approach, as a rebellion against our own upbringing, is common. I meet many women who keep their own mothers at arm's length most of the time, but especially around the time of the birth of a baby. Becoming a mother can throw our own childhoods into stark relief.

'I realised I didn't like the way my mum parented, and although I respect her for all her hard work, we are very, very different mothers.' Emily

'Having her around is useful and it's often nice to chat, but I don't ask her for advice or share much controversial stuff with her because I know, even if she doesn't say it out loud, she's judging me.' Nicole

Another mother tells me:

'People always said to me that having children would change my relationship with my mother for the better as I'd realise what it was like and appreciate her more. Nope. Rather it showed me that she was even more of a shit mother than I already knew and I couldn't believe she'd gone through this process without any self-reflection or attempt to better herself.'

Others may look back with affection on the way their parents brought them up and strive to replicate that approach with their own children. And for some, the experience of childbirth and parenting may deepen the mother-daughter bond, bringing empathy and understanding to a previously fraught or distant relationship.

'Having children of my own was the making of the relationship... Circumstances and events had pushed a crevasse between us from my teens onwards. Becoming a mother made me braver, bolder and willing to face the unspoken. Becoming a

grandmother seemed to pull at her core and together we found a way forward in our relationship.'

'I could not have birthed without my mum there. She just made me feel so safe....Having witnessed me birth my mum immediately became a doula too.' Tamara Cianfini

For a few, the memories of childhood may be raw and painful, but their coping strategy is to tell themselves a story that the suffering was the making of them, that physical punishment 'never did me any harm' or that it 'taught me to respect my elders' or 'made me stronger and more self-reliant'. While I certainly think that human beings are extremely resilient, and children especially so, we are learning that a high-stress environment in the early years can predispose children to living their whole lives flooded with cortisol – in a perpetual 'fight, flight or freeze' state. Chronic stress, associated as it is with inflammation and slower healing, is at the root of many health and psychological issues. Society encourages us to make our own parenting choices, to subcontract our parenting out to nurseries and childminders, and does everything it can to force mothers out of the home. But it is an undeniable truth that the formative years are crucial time when children need at least one anchoring, consistent, responsive relationship. In other words, neither children nor mothers always ripen most deliciously off the bough.

Because most of us know this, deep in our hearts, healing the wounds of our own childhoods often becomes key to the search for how to be mothers ourselves. Some find they need to pick at the scabs, uncovering the depth and profundity of the wound in order to understand it and heal. For others, reaching a state of acceptance and giving themselves permission to move on and find a way to parent that includes self-love is what takes the heat out of the perpetual doubt that plagues them. Whatever happens, our relationship with our own parents, in particular our mothers, is what informs our experience of motherhood beyond all else.

It can feel impossible to let go of the notion that our parents should be everything to us: perfection personified, the be-all and end-all. I have watched so many women use their mothering journey as a love letter, or a slap in the face, to their own mothers – a way to honour or criticise the past. But our parents can never be everything. As writer and mother Susan Mildenhall says, the moment she looked at her parents and asked herself what *one thing* she received from each of her parents, was the day her relationship with them began to fully mature.

If your mother has one thing to teach you, you are blessed. Perhaps it is time to let the other stuff go. Is it really useful or therapeutic to pick at the negatives: the betrayals, the loss or the grief? Or is it time to concentrate on extracting each drop of joy that every passing moment gives us? Each second of clarity, each true human connection, each empathic experience or wise setting of boundaries is a cause for celebration and a reason to be proud.

Perhaps, to accept ourselves as mothers – as parents – we need to accept the way we were parented. This may lead to a more positive relationship with our own parents, but equally it might result in a healthy stepping away and letting go. You will know.

There is no doubt that for many women, motherhood is both a liberation and an imprisonment. On one hand, birth and the act of mothering can be a catalyst for growth, aspiration and inspiration; a time to learn our strengths, the unique gift women have to create and sustain life and to revel in the pride that power brings us. Rather than finding our biology reductionist and restrictive, motherhood sometimes presents a woman with a first experience of awe and pride in her body. If only those caring for us always shared that awe, instead of assuming our bodies are flawed and broken.

'I was 36! Thirty-six! Everyone knows there is a time bomb in a woman's uterus which explodes when she is about 36 and turns her from fecund to mummified cow.' Glee Huntsman

Parenting can teach us that, despite the hard daily grind, which can seem such a thankless task at times, we raise decent kids. Our pride in that achievement should be immense and can lead to new-found confidence, creativity and passions.

Mothers are, in many respects, revered; the ideal mother-figure is still on her pedestal – patient, stoical, never-complaining, ever-loving and nurturing, she heals the woes of the world. For many men, the Perfect Mother on her pedestal is to be respected, yet the same woman, without her child, can be leered at and abused:

'I'm not a mother yet, but most of the time, out and about with babies I take care of, I'm perceived as such. I often experience that with a baby or small child wrapped up on my back/chest I don't get catcalled – but on the way home from work, wearing the same clothes, men do shout sexist shit to me. Once I had a baby on my back, and a guy 'complimented' me on my legs – he didn't see the baby. When we passed by and he realized I 'had' a child, he ran up to me and excused himself.' Sarolta Kremmer

Yet we are imprisoned by social expectations of motherhood. Just as all women are trapped in the patriarchal notions of the dichotomy of the virgin and the whore, mothers are held back, wings clipped, by the simplistic idea that, if the perfect mother falls off her pedestal, she is single-handedly responsible for everything that is wrong with society. Juvenile crime?

Blame the mother – shouldn't she know where her kids are? Drug addiction? Teenage pregnancy? Open any newspaper or magazine and the examples of mother-blame are easy to find.

The dawning realisation that we can, and often are, held accountable for all the ills of society can have a profound effect on a woman's sense of self. Many of us can remember feelings of panic and shame as our babies cried in public or the low moments sitting in toilets or dusty corners feeding hungry babies. Whether the disapproving stares and tuts are imagined or not, the discomfort felt by many women when we fear our parenting or the space we take up as mothers is being judged is tangible. I still blush at the memory of being admonished in the ladies toilets of a shopping centre. I couldn't work out how to pee with my baby in a buggy. I couldn't fit the buggy in the cubicle with me and I was scared to close the door and leave him outside. With rising panic and bursting bladder, I finally sat and peed with the door open, only to be shouted at by a middle-aged woman for exposing myself and blocking the way with my pram.

Whether the judgement is real, or perceived, makes no difference. To me, if a mother is worried about being judged, that fear must be based on something – some unconscious messages she has been receiving about what is, and is not, expected and tolerated.

> 'I remember very clearly the first time I went out with my first baby, in a pram. I was so aware that whereas a few days earlier people would look at me and my bump with a smile and a gentle look, helping me, moving out of the way, I suddenly felt I was being tutted at for taking up pavement space!' Justine Fieth

On top of the normal challenges of new parenthood, many women feel under immense pressure to 'get back to normal'.

This strange phenomenon can take many forms, from an expectation of being back in the size 10 skinny jeans a week after birth, to pressure from employers that ranges from subtle messages that motherhood should not impact on our productivity, to overt signals that mothers are not welcome in the workplace. Think the days of mothers being hounded out of the workplace are over? The days of female nurses and teachers being sacked the moment they got married may be long gone, but I have lost count of the clients I've had who have been overlooked for promotion, undermined, manoeuvred sideways or even made redundant while on maternity leave. For many women, the process of going through a tribunal as a new mother is just too expensive and exhausting, so employers are not held to account.

It seems children are seen as disabling to women in a way that doesn't seem to be the case for men. Hard-won measures to support mothers are usually wishy-washy and diluted by the time they become legislation: many of my clients tell me that they ask to go back to work part-time but are denied by their employers, who are under no legal obligation to acquiesce to the request. Job-sharing is still quite rare. And women are not supported by society to step away from work outside the home, at least for the pre-school years, to concentrate on the important and often fulfilling (and yes, bloody tough) job of bringing up kids. Rather than it being seen as a vital role, 'stay-at-home-mums' are too often portrayed as a drain on society, benefit-scroungers or worse.

'I thought I'd easily be back at work when M was 6 months. [I was] very career orientated, travelled a lot for work, but we were still too interdependent and me too exhausted to contemplate it. I didn't feel up to it.' Ellen Thornhill

One of the first realisations that comes with a baby is that motherhood makes us invisible. Where once I had felt the discomfort of men's eyes following me in the street and endured comments and wolf-whistles on a regular basis, now I felt as though I'd been given Harry Potter's cloak of invisibility. Doors were closed in my face, I was ignored in shops and forgotten in plans for social events. I stood outside shops and at the bottom of flights of steps while people whizzed past on their busy way. I once sat on the floor of a crowded supermarket, next to my tantruming toddler, and tried to conceal my tears by pretending to be extremely interested in breakfast cereal. People stepped over us.

What with the white noise of social judgement and well-meaning advice ringing in the ears of new mothers, it's hardly surprising that so many women are finding it tough to harness their instincts. What do I mean by that? I suppose what I've come to realise is that the knowledge of how to mother – communicating with babies, children and teenagers, loving, comforting and catering for their needs – is pretty much inbuilt. There are some learned skills in the mix, for which we need good modelling and useful guidance from more experienced mothers and well-versed 'experts', but at a deep, primal level, there is a solid, trustworthy voice at the heart of all of us; bred in over millennia, if only we can hear it.

It sometimes feels like the white noise is drowning out everything else. The mothers I meet are often mired in the minutiae of conflicting, bizarre advice from parenting gurus. Baby not sleeping? You're doing it wrong: too many blankets/ not enough blankets. To swaddle or not to swaddle? To feed on a schedule or 'on demand'? Toddler having meltdowns? Is it time to take control, instigate the naughty step and lay down some immutable boundaries to show her who's boss, or try to gently and patiently show empathy and validate those powerful emotions? Whatever we do, apparently we are making a 'rod for our own back' and spoiling the child rotten. The breast that tingles when a baby cries, the heart that hurts when a child is upset, the arms that yearn to hold a child and understand his pain – these parenting reflexes are ignored and subsumed in the abiding cultural meme that kids are merely puppies that need taming.

The emotional landscape inside a child's head is as rich, complex and ever-changing as an adult's. Yet most of my clients seem to be receiving the message that adult emotions deserve to be heard, but a child's do not. Apparently, babies need to be trained to sleep, trained to defecate, trained to defer gratification and encouraged to repress their emotions. The idea that a small person's feelings are as valuable and deserving of validation as an adult's is a revolutionary idea that never seems to make it into the mainstream parenting manuals. Just like our Victorian great-grandparents, it seems we still expect a quiet life and our children to be seen but not heard.

At least that's the idea we have served up to us, often by people who are in positions of authority or expertise. Many doctors, midwives, health visitors and children's centre workers don't appear to be able to guide us with evidence-based information on parenting. My clients are often presented with a *fait accompli*: either you teach babies and children with the carrot and stick method, or you ignore the 'bad' behaviour entirely, withholding love and comfort until the child conforms. Very rarely are parents told it is OK to hold their child, ask how they feel, seek to understand those feelings and hold the space for those feelings to play out in a safe and loving environment. From a baby who craves a mother's warm body throughout the night, to a teenager who needs to rail at the world for a while, to a partner who is frustrated by a work project, we all need to be held, heard, comforted and reassured. A baby's emotional needs are more visceral, immediate and enormous than an adult's, yet we are told they do not count for as much and must be ignored in order to teach them who's boss.

There is something I am noticing as a doula. A growing generalised anxiety, prickling away at women like a nettle sting, keeping them awake, causing obsessive compulsive thoughts or crippling confusion. My clients are increasingly coming home from hospital carrying the heavy weight of all this conflicting advice. They are coming into parenthood weighed down by a feeling that, unless they do everything 'right', they will be *bad* parents. Today, I watched a mother's eyes flick towards the cot. The baby was wriggling, grunting and turning her face towards her mother. Next to the cot stood the grandmother, arms folded, determined look in her eyes. An abiding faith in the inbuilt abilities of parents to follow their instincts is disappearing. We are forgetting to tell parents they are *enough*.

Rather than supporting those who are struggling, we are demonising them. We are forgetting to remind parents that children just need love. And most importantly, as a society, we have forgotten that, in order to give love, parents need to receive it.

Conversely, we are fed another powerful message: that a 'happy mummy' leads to happy children. While on one level this is perfectly true – parental mental health problems or domestic abuse are undoubtedly damaging to kids – this 'advice' over-simplifies matters. On one hand, it implies that nothing we do has any effect on the child, which if it were true would mean that all the psychologists and child development researchers have got it oh-so-wrong and we can go ahead and outsource our parenting to the lowest bidder. On the other hand it gives us absolutely no guidance on *how* to be happy. How *do* we find personal fulfilment in motherhood? How do we learn what we need to be happy, healthy parents; to find our personal balance, our personal space and time to develop ourselves as humans as well as mothers?

In this landscape of censure and reproach, perhaps we must learn to judge ourselves and each other by a new and different set of rules – not by the state of our houses or our ability to 'have it all', not by our kids' abilities to sleep through the night or our commitment to breastfeeding or baby-led weaning or private tutors – but by the small moments of loving touch, the still standing after a rough day, the ability to apologise and reconnect after a temper is lost…

It seems to me that our society has a binary, simplistic notion of motherhood. Tucked away at the fringes are the real, complicated and beautiful realities of the women and men who are working away in the trenches of childcare. Once we begin to understand the normal range of maternal emotion and the real, lived experience of parenthood, perhaps we can then stop judging ourselves and each other and start defining what it is that we need.

Once upon a time, feminists talked about the chains of motherhood, but it is not motherhood per se that imprisons us. It is the social and financial shackles that result in so many of us feeling hampered and held back. Our experience of being daughters and mothers can sometimes prevent us ripening into the juiciest apples; strong and rosy-red and ready to revel in our mothering. Is it too much to dream that women can actually be free to make real, unhindered choices without the ties of money, social expectation and judgement holding us back?

Well, there is always hope. And some small, but real, causes for celebration. The strides we've made, in the last century in particular, have been immense. Improvements in conditions for women and girls around the world have changed the lives of millions. The extremes of poverty and illiteracy affect fewer now than ever before. Recently, the proportion of people living in extreme poverty (subsisting on less than $1.90 per day) fell below 10% for the first time ever. In 1981, it was 44%.

Better housing and sanitation for many women around the world means that losing a child has become a rarity. Whereas once, not too long ago, we could pretty much count on losing one in every three of our children before the age of five, improved public health measures and better nutrition have made an enormous difference. Fewer women in the world grow up stunted by rickets, meaning fewer obstructed labours. Better nutrition has also made us taller and cleverer.

Male doctors finally started washing their hands and stopped moving directly from post-mortem to childbirth in the 1800s, thus putting an end to the epidemic of 'childbed fever' which, in some hospital wards, killed up to 40% of mothers. Since around 1800 the number of children surviving past their fifth birthday has increased exponentially. Today, nearly 96% of the world's children survive infancy, compared to under 57% in 1820.[25]

Freedoms, be they the right to vote, freedom of speech and other kinds of expression, sexuality and access to birth control,* are increasing. There are fewer child marriages, and more and more countries banning FGM.[26]

In the world of education, despite infamous stories of girls and women being denied access to school, things are improving. The Malala Fund is working to get girls more than just a basic, primary education (32 million girls worldwide still miss out on even this).[27]

In the world of birth and parenting, the handful of organisations like AIMS and the White Ribbon Alliance[28] that have valiantly striven to protect and promote maternity rights are now being joined by a swathe of new, energetic and enthusiastic organisations committed to female empowerment and autonomy.

---

* Especially important since we have broken the link between unrestricted, exclusive, full-term breastfeeding and child spacing – yes, it works as well as condoms – look up 'lactational amenorrhea'.

The Red Tent Movement and the Positive Birth Movement are powerful examples of grassroots gatherings of women coming together to support, educate and inform each other.[29] Birthrights is another relatively new organisation founded by birth workers and lawyers that is working to raise awareness of the fact that *'all women are entitled to respectful maternity care that protects their fundamental rights to dignity, autonomy, privacy and equality.'* [30]

Within the doula community, our Access Fund volunteers provide psychosocial support to vulnerable women and families or those who are in financial need. For many, their Access Fund doula is their only source of continuous emotional and practical support through pregnancy, birth and the early days with the new baby. The fund's coordinator, Sarah Stephen-Smith, shared this testimonial from a recipient of the fund:

> *'My pregnancy was spent in a mixed homeless hostel with people battling addictions and mental health issues; although I had support workers and professional help I felt scared and like a patient. The access fund was a lifeline to me providing emotional support and lots of practical information about looking after a baby, and empowering me through a birthing experience which was traumatic, and difficult nursing. It was life-changing to feel that someone was on my side and helping me as an individual rather than a medical charge.'*

Birth Companions, a London-based charity, works with women in prison, providing support through pregnancy and birth.[31] Around the country doulas are working in many different ways in partnership with agencies such as social services and refugee support charities.

2017 marks 60 years since the formation of La Leche League (LLL), the first mother-to-mother breastfeeding support organisation committed to empowering mothers to understand how breastfeeding works so they can help themselves and go on to help others. LLL was soon joined in the UK by the Association of Breastfeeding Mothers (ABM) and Breastfeeding Network (BfN), while the NCT also has a breastfeeding support arm. All run support groups, telephone helplines and training courses, while advocating for breastfeeding to be higher up the political agenda and for the NHS do a better job of supporting mothers to reach their breastfeeding goals.

And then there is social media. It is bringing mothers and those who serve them together as a force for change. Yes, it can be a negative influence; bombarded by images of everyone else's perfect lives, buffeted by negative, aggressive threads about what we should and shouldn't be doing, we can close our feeds feeling like dreadful people and terrible parents. This daily habit could even be undermining of our mental health. But I think the trick is to find our safe spaces of like-minded people and acknowledge that when groups work best, they aren't just gangs of women bigging each other up, but are spaces for lovingly challenging each other and supporting the growth and development of all the other members. Twitter, in particular, seems to be a place where parents, parent-advocates and health workers can meet on a platform of equality and listen and learn from each other. The relationship networks that result are creating magical joint projects and beautiful cross-fertilisation. MatExp,[32] a collaboration of parents, health professionals, lay peer supporters and other interested parties is a good example of this cooperative approach.

Lauren Derrett, author of *Filter Free*, an exploration of the way women use social media, told me about her experience of Facebook as a force for female solidarity:

'Motherhood can be the loneliest place on earth... to get through it with your sanity intact you need to be surrounded

by like-minded women who hear you, empathise with you and above all, support you. In my search for this support I set up my own group on Facebook called We are Enough. We currently have near on 800 women all connecting every day, sharing, laughing, listening and supporting.'

There are hundreds of groups, large and small, with similar aspirations.

In the sphere of reproductive rights there is much great work going on around the world. There is a growing awareness that once we lift women out of poverty and give them free access to education, together with social and political control over their own lives, birth rates drop, thus preventing population pressures on limited resources. Control over fertility, including birth control, support for exclusive breastfeeding and safe abortion would save many thousands of lives every year. Against a backdrop of vociferous opposition to women having dominion over their own fertility, people are fighting, for no reward, to safeguard these fundamental rights, smooth out inequalities and stand up against discrimination of all kinds. Take, for example, the Planned Parenthood escorts, who volunteer to walk with women through crowds of protesters to enter abortion clinics.[33] Or the women of colour and their allies campaigning against the disparities in health care and breastfeeding support.

In my own little corner of the birth world, what gives me hope on a daily basis are the mothers and midwives in partnership, campaigning for choice, respect and continuity of carer in childbirth. The daily tiny actions that add up to a groundswell of change. The people – mothers and midwives – who see a lack of provision, or a need for something, and just get up and start doing something:

'The charity Remember my Baby has photographers who take pictures of parents' last moments with their angel babies. The photographer comes out and takes photos for the family. I had such a cry over this when I learned of it.' J'Nel Metherell

'The NHS maternity staff who put positive family centred experience at the core of their work. The midwifery manager who took the time to go through all the concerns of a mother traumatised by a previous birth. The consultant who walked in and said… "Have you heard of gentle cesareans? It's what I do as standard". The registrar who assisted at his first gentle caesarean and provided... respectful care postnatally.' Lindsey Middlemiss

'Airedale Hospital HoM Mary Armitage and Deputy HoM Sarah Simpson for having the vision and foresight to support the Yorkshire Storks IMs.' Millicent Bystander

'A 44-year-old woman supported in her home birth choice when her baby had Down Syndrome and when that baby died, the midwives who were with her when she birthed her baby in water by candlelight, and told her it was one of the most beautiful births they had seen. And the midwives who came to her baby's funeral and hugged her and came to her house and cried. And laughed and gave her hope for the future.' Victoria Greenly

In the last five years there has been an explosion of mother-to-mother support. Sling libraries, small charities that provide baby equipment to families in need, breastfeeding peer support schemes, doulas extending the hand of friendship to women in challenging circumstances. Online groups offering peer support for everything from breech babies to birth after to caesarean, parenting forums and maternity rights. There are people who campaign for equality of provision and more respectful care for groups that have traditionally been ignored. For example, women from minority ethnic groups have consistently been found to be *'less likely to feel spoken to so they could understand, to be treated with kindness, to be sufficiently involved in decisions and to have confidence and trust in the staff.*[34] Birth trauma victims, abuse survivors and those suffering from mental health problems are slowly being recognised as having distinct, complex needs in maternity care and throughout their parenting lives and work is being done in some places to improve services with all minority groups in mind.

There is still much to be done. Good practice still too often stays in little pockets and doesn't spread. There is too little networking and sharing of best practice. It must not be forgotten that much of the grassroots support for families is filling gaps created by wholesale cuts to services for young families or, in some countries, the complete absence of state provision. War and his brothers Starvation and Migration stop so many improvements in their tracks.

I might be blind and stupid, but I choose to have hope and a faith in humanity. I choose to trust that women and birthing people will find how to birth and parent in ways that are healthy and happy for them. I choose to believe that humanity will come to see that we need to look after the Motherhood Tree. Her strong branches and deep roots are what sustain us all. Her shade, her strong trunk to lean on, her beautiful blossom and bountiful fruit must be protected and nurtured. In a million ways, in a million places, people are stepping up to do just that.

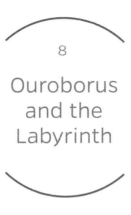

8

Ouroborus and the Labyrinth

'*A woman's psychic and physical journey from maidenhood to motherhood during pregnancy, labor, and postpartum, is surely labyrinthine.*'

Pam England

Every time I sit in a group of aspiring doulas I ask them if they know the difference between a labyrinth and a maze. It is rare that anyone knows the answer. Most of us know, however, that a maze is a puzzle. Something to be figured out. Walking a maze means we are in constant danger of getting lost or trapped in a dead-end. A labyrinth, however, is a single path that merely needs to be followed in order to reach the centre. It may twist and turn, sometimes feeling like it takes us further away from our goal, but all that is required is trust, determination and a commitment to put one foot in front of the other.

A wise and wonderful old woman once told me that doulas are mother-whisperers. Like a volatile and skittish colt, a pregnant woman is easily spooked. Her ears are wide open to horror stories, her heart and womb are opening to make way for the baby and she can be vulnerable to less-than-helpful words and actions and feel trapped in a maze, unsure of which direction to take. She is so soft and exposed at this time, that a brusque word or a lack of empathy will cut her to the quick and probably be remembered forever. All her millions of nerve-endings are at the surface, exposed and exquisitely sensitive; the look in an eye, the twitch of an eyebrow or the curve of a lip may send her into paroxysms of agony and self-doubt. It is earth-shatteringly easy to turn the labyrinth into a maze.

What an impact a friendly companion, who cares only about the emotional state of the person she is supporting, can have! With kind eyes, and soft words she has a magical, calming effect. What are you doing when you listen to a traumatic birth story or a tale of breastfeeding woe or a worry about a child being bullied at school? Is there a value in honouring the story? I think so. Mothers' stories are mainly hidden and forgotten. I have been told birth stories by 80-year-old grandmothers. Every one of the hundreds of women who have attended my doula course has written their birth and early parenting stories. No one has been unable to find the words. The stories are often long and detailed, and it is not uncommon for the act of writing to release long-suppressed emotions.

Being truly heard and validated has a profoundly therapeutic effect. Listening can help a mother fall back in love with her baby, or begin to for the first time, releasing her instincts and allowing her hormones to flow. And we mustn't forget the partner-whispering – they are on a journey too. In fact the whole family is undergoing a transformation as each child arrives.

Parenting in the 21st century can seem more of a maze than a labyrinth – something to be figured out, solved and understood. Questions about roles, gender identities and nature v nurture are more, not less, complicated and confusing than when our grandparents were raising their kids. We are living and loving in uncertain times, with new family structures and attitudes towards parenting becoming more visible than ever before. Our thinking can get caught in cul-de-sacs as we muddle our way through the maze of conflicting opinion and furious words on social media. Meanwhile, the world tries to put us into clearly delineated groups and pit us against each other.

I started this book by offering up a theory that mothering is a verb, not a noun – a word of doing rather than being, action rather than state. But I'm not sure it's that simple.

It is a question that ignites fires in bellies and sparks long, passionate threads on the internet. It touches on how we define ourselves as individuals and feeds into our perception of the society and culture we belong to. As the shapes and sizes of our families adapt and morph in response to seismic shifts in the world, the way we view mothering and the words we use to define it inevitably change too.

I have supported many families that do not conform to the traditional ideas of the nuclear family. I have encountered many ways of describing the parenting roles. There is a beautiful fluidity and freedom to today's families and the ways they choose to express their identities that I love, and which I truly believe are just as likely to produce psychologically healthy children as any other kind of family. Yet these families still encounter prejudice and discomfort.

'I feel like I understand privilege in a lived way – I have been for society [both] gay and straight – I've walked both of those walks and it's easier when you're straight. It's just a smoother ride.' Anon

What are your opinions about biology, gender and parenting? We have certainly grown beyond the socially restrictive attitudes that a family should be made up of a man and a woman, married with kids, with the father working outside and the mother inside the home, thank goodness. What do you believe a child needs to grow and flourish?

Nick, a father in Cambridge, took over the daily care of his baby from when his daughter was six months old. It made financial sense for his wife to go back to full-time work and for Nick to be at home. When I asked him what he felt about gender and parenting, he told me:

> *'I don't believe in mothering, or fathering, just good parenting. I don't think gender has much to do with whether people are good parents or not. [To] attach gender roles to parenting is like trying to attach gender roles to other things, like employment – it can lead to discrimination.'*

I admire his determination to bring his daughter up without gender-orientated restrictions. The choices this family have made during their daughter's formative years are certainly working well for them. I wonder, though, if we are quite ready for a blindness to gender in the parenting sphere. Denying biology, when it comes to parenting, runs the risk of erasing some positives despite laudable attempts to smooth out inequalities. Try as we might, we cannot escape the realities of nature – it is the birthing person who grows the child in a uterus and makes milk for the baby. Many of us would not want to escape that reality, even if we could; although delighting in our biology, revelling in the superpowers nature has given us and enjoying the pleasures our bodies can give us is something that society has determinedly closed its eyes and ears to.

Until society is truly inclusive, we can't be blind to our differences. Black and ethnic minority women still encounter disparities in the quality of the maternity care they receive, feeling less cared for and less likely to have 'satisfactory experiences of pregnancy, childbirth and the postnatal period'.[35]

So many of us need a little more awareness from society and some special provision from others to make us comfortable. Just as in other spheres of life, along with equality, we need to celebrate diversity. Aiming for equity of opportunity, rather than blindly talking about equality, seems vital. Sometimes, some people need an extra helping hand to access the same opportunities as everyone else. Not because they are inherently less able, but because the conditions for them to thrive do not exist. The hurdles have been there for so long, they can be hard to spot.

I wonder too, if being blind to our differences inadvertently erases the history and suffering so many women have endured. Denying differences is easy if you are the one with privilege. It's not so easy when you are the one being discriminated against. For example, being blind to sex and gender may result in a trans man being treated insensitively during pregnancy and birth by health professionals who thoughtlessly call him a woman. Being blind to our differences may result in a pregnant woman losing her job or missing out on a promotion. It may restrict a woman's choice to breastfeed until her child is ready to wean, or result in her being judged and punished for desiring to stay at home with her preschoolers. Being blind to gender prevents us seeing the very real discrimination that women and mothers currently face, and it stops us opening up access to opportunities and choices for all.

Mothers manifest in many forms. Before having my own kids, I became a step-mother, living with my wonderful stepson. I was young, and I had to work out from scratch how to approach the role and make our blended family work. I had no role models and no guidance, other than my instinct and genuine love for him. My lovely boy is now in his 30s and I think things have moved on; judgement of step-families is less negative and society is a little more inclusive.

For lesbian co-mothers, their transition to motherhood

may very much depend on the way they are treated by others and when and how they have their children. If the families of non-birth mothers do not accept them as parents, or their identities are questioned by health professionals or antenatal teachers, they can struggle to step into a role as co-parent and suffer psychologically. Being a parent in a same-sex relationship can often be plain sailing these days, but it can sometimes present very real parenting challenges. Kate Edwards, a mother of four, told me

'...people have been quite hurtful... "Why did you have children if you knew you were gay?"... "Why did you get married?" "How do your kids feel?" All these direct and personal questions that straight people don't have to answer. My ex-husband at the time of our separation used my sexuality and coming out as a way to tell me and others that I was unfit to be a mother... He was horrified that they in turn might "turn out gay"... there is still tension and I feel sorry for our children that they have had to listen to anti-gay conversations when they spend time with him.'

Jo Stratford, who has raised her children for many years in a lesbian co-parenting family structure, mused on her particular anxieties about male input into her children's upbringing.

'I've always been looking for the male role model because I have believed children need positive male exemplars. When I told my son I was a lesbian, he said "Oh no!" I thought it was about me being gay but actually, at the age of six, he was worried about having yet another woman in the house as well as his mum and sisters. Even at that young age he was yearning for male energy. I do wonder, though, whether me looking outward for that male input impacted on my mothering...'

During my time as a doula I have been honoured to spend time with lesbian co-parents, adoptive mothers and mothers who have been supported by surrogacy. The beautiful spectrum of emotions they experience when a child joins the family is no different to biological mothers. They feel the same love, the same fierce protective instinct, the same confusion and overwhelm. There is nothing morally superior to biological motherhood. We all walk the same parenting labyrinth. And just like everyone else, sometimes the way ahead looks clear and sometimes the path meanders or menacingly seems to travel away from the goal.

I have also known many women who are parenting alone, through circumstance or by choice. It can be undeniably hard: on a practical level, with no one else to share the burdens of care, on a financial level, juggling work and childcare on one income and on a social level, feeling that all the ills of society are blamed on single mothers. If you have children young *and* you are single, then according to the tabloid newspapers you are a benefit-scrounging, drug-addled drain on society. Add being a woman of colour into that mix and everyday life can be challenging indeed.

'Being a single mother is a blessing in so many ways. I get to sail the mothership with my rules, my sensitivities, my heart... It feels so freeing, asserting and empowering to make all the decisions, small and big. The biggest drawback is how relentless it is to nurture two little souls while trying to nurture mine too. While I crave five minutes of peace, I feel so lucky to feel emotionally supported by my friends. It has led us to have a richer life full of role models.' Lorette Michellon

Sometimes, single motherhood is a consequence of escape and is therefore a celebration of freedom:

'I was horribly abused by her father and that abuse escalated and continued to her. I am so lucky he died because the abuse stopped and the division he was trying to create between

us evaporated... Now I feel the ease of just being with her, educating her, being myself... This new life we have together is amazing.' Abigail Peck

If mothering is a verb, can anyone do it? I certainly think there are aspects of mothering that, when brought into a caring role, are life-enhancing and altogether positive. Jo Gough, a doula, shared her thoughts with me as she mused on the question of whether 'mother' is a verb or a noun.

'I am not a mother. I have no children. But I do mother; I nurture, love boundlessly and fiercely, I comfort and hold. These are all aspects of mothering... It makes me reflect on my doula role, am I seen as less legit given I'm not a mother? Can I "mother a mother" without an experience of mothering? How much of my work as a doula is driven by my own loss of mother, and the unfulfilled need I had as a young woman to be mothered in the way I do for others now?'

And of course, not all women wish to be mothers. The reasons why are varied and complex.

Feminist academic Dr Anija Dokter thinks:

'it's also a deep ecological consciousness. So many babies are born in situations of rape, coercion, duty, requirement, slavery... babies born for other people, out of expectation and sometimes even for survival's sake (I've just been reading stories about women who were set on fire by their families for being barren or giving birth to girls). What if women only had the babies they truly wanted for themselves? This would require a cultural revolution so that sexual and reproductive consent is truly possible. I deeply believe that, if this were the case, we would have a fraction of the population boom and ecological disasters we are facing today. I have seen women have various responses to this sense of ecological disaster for their own

bodies and the world around them. Some women want to bear children powerfully as a way of resisting (like the woman who birthed at the frontlines of the DAPL protest), and some want to say no to the whole thing. Both are beautiful responses.'

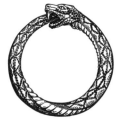 Here I come, right back round in a circle, to wonder again, what is mothering? Where does it come from? Is it dependent on biology? It seems to me, the more I look at mothering, the more it reminds me of the ancient mythical creature, the Ouroborus, the famous snake swallowing its own tail – an ancient symbol of introspection and the eternal cycle of life: birth, death, destruction and rebirth. Ouroborus eats its own tail to survive, in an eternal cycle of regeneration. Just like the snake shedding its skin, mothers reinvent themselves in a perpetual cycle of growth and renewal. Just as we adapt to the phase our children are going through, they change, and we must morph again in response. Mothering is something and everything, all-encompassing or just part of who we are. It is biology fulfilling a primal drive, but also a feeling, an activity independent of who we are, how we identify, and our life choices.

Mothering, says Emma, is both:

'a noun and a verb. Maybe in the sense that I mother my son when I am with him, but my identity is now fully entwined with that so even when I'm not mothering I am still a mother. I don't believe mother has anything to do with sexuality, but sex and gender play a role. Watching the girls at nursery you can already see a mothering tendency; whether that has come from nurture or nature is hard to say.'

Some delight in their biology, while for others, their bodies seem to betray them or become the enemy. While sometimes the roles we inhabit feel comfortable and secure, sometimes to fully express themselves and raise their children in the way they feel right, mothers may need to push back against strict social attitudes or ideas. Many of us are prevented from fully expressing our mothering, tied down and restricted by lack of money and opportunity, sexual or racial discrimination or social isolation.

But at the root of all of us, is mother. Ouroborus, 'one is all', keeper of the kundalini energy, the power of fertility and enlightenment. At the heart of the Ouroborus is infinity; born as women are, with the eggs that can become our future children already nestled within us. The snake eats its own tail; immortal and endless.

We are, I hope, able to be unified by the one, universal and inescapable fact that all of us – every single human being – once floated, warm and safe, in a dark, wet womb. Almost all of us had a very first, primal experience of love in the arms of a mother and I don't see this state of affairs changing any time soon. What we must change, though, is a world that uses a woman's ability to gestate and give birth as an excuse to vilify and oppress her. The bodies of women, and mothers in particular, have long been battlegrounds: patriarchy is played out in our wombs, breasts, hearts and minds. As the great Adrienne Rich says so eloquently in her book *Of Woman Born*: *'The body has been made so problematic for women that it has often seemed easier to shrug it off and travel as a disembodied spirit.'*

I was sold the lie as an undergraduate in Women's Studies class that my liberation is as a 'disembodied spirit'. The Pill, sexual freedom, a career, no kids, or at least kids that didn't interrupt my career trajectory, was my destiny. And liberation from my body was my only chance at equality. I have come to believe that modern feminism needs to be a whole lot more encompassing of the many flavours of womanhood if we are to get anywhere. To be truly intersectional, we're going to have to face some tough questions. But if we can't accept and forgive each other, Ouroborus will devour itself.

There is biological magic in motherhood; the DNA we inherit and pass on, together with our antibodies, the amazing good bacteria of our microbiome, our breastmilk, our hormones. It is an undeniably powerful chemical soup; one that can be both enrapturing and traumatic to bathe in. But there are other kinds of just-as-wonderful magic. Oxytocin binds us as families whatever form that family takes. All parents need, and usually display, immense patience, creativity, fortitude and stoicism as well as fathomless love. Families are made and function well when there is love, commitment and empathic, responsive parenting. When communities, neighbours and friends support each other. When fathers, partners, grandparents, aunts and uncles all feed into a child's growth and development. The beautiful strands of love and caring work a child needs to thrive are not confined to a biological mother.

This work of caring – the daily grind of seeing the sunrise with a early-rising toddler, changing nappies, cooking a meal the whole family will eat, doing the jigsaw, reading the Gruffalo for the millionth time, pacing the floorboards at 3am with a crying baby, weathering the emotional storm because you gave a child the wrong colour cup or the broccoli is touching the potatoes – is relentless, and hard, and wonderful. It is at once profound and mundane. These are the little actions that measure out our lives. They are the steps on the labyrinth. Part of this journey is about trusting the path, having faith in our travelling companions and remembering to slow down, taking each twist and turn in the route mindfully; consciously focusing on where we are now, not where we are going or where we have come from. It is the here and now that matters in parenting. All those tiny moments, those fleeting interactions, the getting it right and feeling good, and the getting it wrong, saying sorry and moving on. All too often we are left, travelling the labyrinth alone, trailing the kids behind us, in a hurry to reach the end. So many of us lack travelling companions; the partners, parents, extended family, neighbours and friends that once spread the load and made raising children less energy-sapping and more fun.

When we have companions on the path, children receive their birthright – to just come along for the ride. It doesn't seem like much, but the gifts of learning and education that children receive from being alongside us, experiencing the world and all its challenges and opportunities through the eyes of a guardian adult and from the safe haven of loving arms, are what allow a child to manage their emotions and take their place in society. Children want to see us live, laugh, love, work and wander through the labyrinth of life. They want to come along in-arms and then trot along beside us, dragging their heels behind us and running far ahead. They need to be able to return to their centre; the beating heart of their world, their first love, and sip from the mothering cup when they are hurt or emotionally wounded. In this way, parenting is nothing special and simultaneously precious beyond price.

This shared journey allows adults to spread their wings and have the physical energy, emotional resilience and the creative drive to do other things. When the basics of life are catered for, that is when mothers can express themselves. It is no coincidence that I wrote my first book when my youngest child was 11. With no parenting help beyond my husband, and the financial imperative to work pretty much full-time, my creative urges were curtailed. It makes me wonder how much talent, creativity and invention we are missing out on by ensuring women are trapped doing the majority of the childrearing on top of being tied to jobs they often don't enjoy.

What talents and achievements we bring to the world when we have time! With psychosocial support networks, enough to eat, financial stability and some education, women can change the world! Parenthood brings many of the superpowers needed for achievement, including a driving need to protect and provide for our offspring and new, creative, energy-efficient ways of thinking laterally that often result in beautiful new solutions to age-old problems.

Even Mary Wollstonecraft, early feminist writer, born in 1759, recognised that women can be bound and gagged by marriage and children when they do not have freedom of thought and expression:

> 'To be a good mother — a woman must have sense, and that independence of mind which few women possess who are taught to depend entirely on their husbands.'

I increasingly see families rearranging themselves in complex and endlessly creative ways in order to give everyone an income and fulfilment through personal expression. We take risks, giving up secure jobs to set up our own businesses or pursue the education or career we dream of. We use our skills, both new and ancient, to keep the wolf from the door, and our creations are often beautiful as well as useful. We take the time to care for those who cannot care for themselves – the young, the sick and the old. Lift us just a little bit out of grinding poverty and we add enormously to the sum of human happiness. We can create life and sustain it with a liquid from our breasts that protects against disease as well as nourishes our children. And yet most of this work is never counted in the worth of a civilization or included in the calculations of Gross National Product.

I asked my friends and colleagues to tell me about women they admire and the outpouring was overwhelming and inspiring: from Joan of Arc to Maya Angelou, Marie Curie and Frida Kahlo, through to modern public figures fighting injustice, like Thabitha Khumalo. Yet many admitted that the very first woman who came to mind was their mother or influential mother-figure from their childhood.

'Mrs Seredyn – my teacher. She believed in me...and was my first role model. She listened when others didn't. She showed how clearly she deeply cared about all her students.' Zoe Walsh

'My mum, who is a tough old bird.' Karen Hall

So where are we going? What will we find in the centre of the labyrinth? What lies waiting for us in the future? I wish I were clever enough to have any real insights into the future of gender and parenting politics. I do know what I wish for my daughter: that she have the freedom to choose what she does with her body and when. That she has the right to loving, skilled healthcare and emotional support through the transitions of life. That she has a voice that is heard and freedom to use her brain and talents to express her unique qualities. I know she can't 'have it all' and that she will sometimes need to make tough choices, but I want those choices to be hers, and hers alone, not dictated by the endless hunger of capitalism or the power-crazed needs of the patriarchy. If she decides to have children, I hope she has social support so she can enjoy them without having to choose between spending time with them, or feeding and clothing them. And I hope she can co-parent with the person she loves, without judgement or ridicule and that she feels able to teach her children that they deserve the same rights. I dream of her walking the labyrinth, not trapped in the dead ends of the maze.

I do know this about the centre of the labyrinth: is a celebration, a remembering and a breather before the onward journey. It is a moment for reflection on how far we've come and a reminder not to stop striving for our rights. Now is not the time to rest on our laurels or take our gains and privileges for granted. Because, as the inspirational Malala Yousafzai says, *'We realize the importance of our voices only when we are silenced.'*

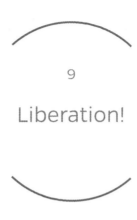

9

Liberation!

'To nourish children and raise them against odds is in any time, any place, more valuable than to fix bolts in cars or design nuclear weapons.'

Marilyn French

During the writing of this book I have, I admit, been struggling. The challenges have been multiple, but it feels like every knock has chipped off another unnecessary part of me and honed my thinking; simplifying things in a very organic way.

First, the inspirational Vanessa Olorenshaw published *Liberating Motherhood* – the book I wanted to write but knew, deep in my bones, I couldn't. The book that is the political treatise I have been yearning for; the call to action, the simple explanation of why I, and so many mothers I meet, feel disenfranchised, discriminated against and forgotten. Vanessa, I thank you. Your book, and the accompanying Purple Stockings campaign will go down in history, taught in Women's Studies seminars alongside What Women Want, the Red Stockings movement and the Million Women Rising. You made me realise that it is OK to be smaller, and more personal, because the personal *is* the political. All of us, as individuals, make up society, and it is women sharing their personal narratives that galvanises us and helps us make sense of the world.

Second, as I was struggling to write, I watched as the world seemed to go mad and bad and downright atrocious, towards women and people of colour in particular. I watched as the children of Syria were bombed out of their homes. I cried as I watched refugees arriving in vast numbers on the shores of Europe. I moaned in disbelief when early attempts to help and support them dwindled and our governments appeared to ignore the crisis. I held my head in my hands as, around the world, people began to vote for isolationism; denying our global village and our collective responsibility for each other. I gasped as I watched a man who boasted about abusing women and denying human rights to whole segments of the population win the US presidency and close the US borders. It felt like everything we had worked so hard for was being dismantled.

In the same week as Trump was elected, I went to the refugee camp in Dunkirk. I needed to see with my own eyes. What I witnessed there crystallised everything I had been feeling and everything I have been trying to explore in this book. I saw human suffering in the raw, and who suffered most? Mothers and children. Confined to cold, damp shacks as soon as it got dark, or somehow trying to work out how to smuggle small children over the water to the UK, families huddle together, feeling hopeless and friendless. Mothers are often separated from their children – imprisoned for protesting against the harsh treatment of the French authorities. I saw mothers struggling with the behaviour of their traumatised children, and mothers unable to be emotionally available to their children because of their own trauma. And I saw mothers and babies who are well attached and loving and doing their best, in appalling conditions.

I saw how the well-meaning but ill thought-out actions of those who want to help can have dangerous ramifications for the most vulnerable: donations of out-of-date baby milk powder, cartons that had been opened months before and brands that are not designed to be given to babies were rife in the camp. Bottles and teats were being handed out on request, despite the fact that there were few facilities for washing and sterilising the equipment. The volunteers had little understanding that possibly contaminated powdered formula increases the risk of illness and potentially death for small babies.

Mothers are giving birth in conditions that threaten their physical and mental health every day. In rich countries and poor countries, the care a woman can expect to receive may not be appropriate to her needs. My friend and fellow doula, Lisa Sykes, tells me that refugee women in Greece are almost always given caesarean sections, denied the right to be accompanied by their husbands and sent back to the camp with formula milk, because many doctors are apparently under the misapprehension that stressed mothers will need to formula feed. Treating women this way causes suffering for the men, too: separated from their wives or shouldering the burdens of care and worry on top of all the privations they are already enduring.

This year I have seen up close what happens when women have to cope with the fallout. War, poverty, violence. Rape, trafficking, crime and domestic abuse. Women and children are always the biggest victims. Mothers are always the most vulnerable, being least able to fend for themselves while caring for small children.

I began to see that motherhood is a litmus test for a society: measure how well treated the mothers are in a particular time and place and it will tell you all you need to know about the way that society regards its most vulnerable citizens and what value it places on raising the next generation of emotionally rounded, mentally healthy people. People likely to love and support their neighbours. People who are unlikely to punch each other or drop bombs on babies.

In times of peace and prosperity, it is easy for mothers to be blind to the privations and challenges that patriarchy heaps on motherhood. Many of us have been handed the crumbs of male privilege and it has shut us up; careers, the right to vote and our fragile right to control our own fertility have sold us the lie that feminism is no longer needed: we have won equality, if we want it. If you don't, stay at home with the brats.

But increase poverty, allow unequal access to birth control, education and financial support and choice becomes a thing of the past. The suffering of women and mothers increases exponentially. And history does not always move inexorably toward a brighter future; in the US today some states are attempting to legislate against abortion and restrict a woman's right to control her own fertility.

Heap other forms of privation and discrimination on top and things get silly. Are you a woman of colour? Are you more comfortable in non-binary gender roles or are you gay, queer or bi? Are you struggling with the added challenges of class, access to education or teetering on the poverty line? Then you don't need me, a privileged, middle-class, educated straight-ish white woman to tell you anything about the hardships you face. All I can say is that whether a person wishes to escape their biology or embrace it, our only hope is solidarity, our only means of achieving equity is standing together, working on mutual understanding and giving each other a whole lot of rope when we inevitably mess up, offend each other or grope for meaning in a confusing world. Parenting is tough. As the mother of almost-grown teens, looking back along the long, winding parenting path, I can only tell you my truth: loneliness is no fun, judging and being judged is no fun, cliques and one-upwomanship is no blooming fun at all. Let each other off the hook and offer each other a helping hand because... well, because it makes all the difference to how families feel and how families function.

'I don't know how I would have got through without your kind, listening heart. I lost count of the times you put me at ease and the times you were at the end of the phone…' Katrina

I have spent much of this book marvelling at the majesty of biological motherhood. That is not because I think this form of mothering should take precedence over any other, but because as a doula and breastfeeding counsellor, it is what I see almost every day – women growing and birthing babies and stepping into a world that is new and strange. What I see, for the most part, is that whoever you are, however you identify and whatever your route to parenthood, you are probably not getting the support, validation or the practical help that you need. When it comes to the crucial job of raising the next generation, the playing field is not level.

This book is, at its heart, about choice. And that is because, at my heart, I am a doula and choice is what we are all about. Choice is what gets us all excited and riled up; what we think about when we wake up and as we go to sleep. Choice isn't about being invited to tea, being offered a digestive biscuit and being told to be grateful. It's about being able to peruse the whole selection pack and pick the pink wafer, or the bourbon, or the custard cream because you *like* it, or opt not to eat biscuits at all, without having to justify your preference. Choice is about informed consent and informed refusal – having the freedom to accept or decline what is on offer. Choice is about being respected and accepted, whoever you are and however you decide to manifest your role as parent. Want to get a nanny and go back to work at three months?

Let's work together to make that a happy and healthy transition. Want to freebirth in a yurt, home educate and raise goats? More power to your elbow. All I care about is that you are in possession of your whole menu of options and that you have the practical, emotional and financial support to have true freedom to make the decisions that feel right for you.

I want us to be able to be out and proud about our preferences, and to feel free and liberated enough to do what feels right, for ourselves and our children. Apparently, according to an old English saying, it's a woman's prerogative to change her mind; but I don't see much of a right to make a choice in the first place, let alone the opportunity to change tack as we go along, according to our needs or circumstances. A woman's *needs* are relegated to the list of things we don't talk about, that are not considered important or are vaguely taboo.

Whether in safe, middle-class areas of Europe, or in refugee camps and bombed-out houses, 'women's business' is a phrase that conjures up mumbled whispering behind hands, often accompanied by a male shudder at the thought of inherently female bodily functions and a feeling that the issues that concern women are marginal, unimportant, petty and to be ignored. Subjects that affect women have been ghettoised, as though society needs not to hear about our pains and struggles. Write to the agony aunt in the women's pages of the newspaper. Talk to your gynaecologist. Don't bother *us* with your tribulations. And so women, and mothers in particular, are prevented from bringing their concerns to the attention of wider society.

This makes me furious on a number of levels. For a start, since when is 51% of the population a minority topic? How can the very real challenges that women face be ignored or sidelined? And when did we forget that if something is a problem for women, it's a problem for *all* of us? Women's business is not something that men can ignore. Mothers, carers, nurses and childcarers are

141

almost always women. And these jobs are the cornerstones of a well-functioning, fit-for-purpose society. In fact, society is pretty much built on women's work. *Mothers' work.*

What does it tell us that a woman was summarily dismissed from ever having a chance of becoming prime minister of the UK because she had the temerity to talk about the insight and skills she might have gained from being a mother? Yes, her wording was clumsy, but what have we come to, that talking about the qualities and qualifications that motherhood brings us is so taboo that we must be instantly silenced? Andrea Leadsom, relegated to a footnote in political history for the crime of being proud of being a mother, I have to admit to feeling just a tiny bit sorry for you, even if I would never have voted for you!

At the end of the day, the phrase 'women's business' conjures up far more for me than traditional images of domestic work and sanitary towels. Whether it's nature or nurture, the reality is that, in general, women seem to excel when it comes to work that requires emotional intelligence, empathy, communication skills and relationship-building.

The way women do business, from micro-businesses in Africa and Asia, 'mompreneurs', kitchen-table businesses or the boardroom, the creativity motherhood brings seems to enhance and energise women like nothing else. There is a *focus,* for example, that inevitably comes when our work is encompassed within the boundaries of school runs, which opens up interesting new abilities and opportunities to think outside the box. Women around the world are identifying problems or challenges and finding solutions; creating businesses that fulfil a real need or achieving their dreams. I once supported a single mother, living in one room in university accommodation, to finish her PhD during her postpartum. To give her time to read and write while the baby was asleep, we figured out that putting her laptop on a shelf, so she could stand and sway with her baby in a sling, gave her two hours in the afternoon to work. At other times she cocooned herself in bed, with the baby on the breast, and typed while he fed. Necessity really is the mother of invention.

I think it is because of necessity that we do things differently to men. We tend towards working cooperatively, rather than competitively. Female leaders are everywhere I look, and they are finding ways to reach consensus and building collaboration in the groups they lead. Our creativity tends towards projects that include others, making potential competitors into partners and building long-term relationships with our colleagues and customers. Becoming a mother changes us. It changes our brains, our expectations, our needs, our interests and passions, but most of all I think it just teaches us to get the hell on with it because life isn't a rehearsal.

'I couldn't make myself go back to a career of marketing. It just didn't suit my mindset or ethics anymore, it had all shifted.' J'Nel Metherell

In south Sudan, women run mobile phone charging points. In Britain, we stack shelves in the supermarket or hold down office jobs to pay the rent. Mothers give up successful careers to follow new desires and passions.

'having a baby wasn't going to define or change me… after the birth of my second child [I] left the career that had always been part of my identity… I think having children fundamentally changes us as women in ways that we can't predict or sometimes fully understand!' Sally Golightly

'I swapped being a 16-hour-a-day, super high stress barrister for being a breastfeeding counsellor, charity trustee and lecturer/advocate on human rights in childbirth law. I did four years of full-on mothering without ever missing the stress of my old job (motherhood did transform me), but I desperately

missed the advocacy for those who were in positions of vulnerability and disempowerment. Took me two years of seriously focussing/connecting/building/listening/learning/manifesting, and some serious nudging and encouragement from some extraordinarily special friends, but I now feel I am on the path that I am meant to be on.' Johanna Rhys-Davis

Around the world, mothers are mobilising. In the face of an inexorable lurch to the political right and greater draconian measures against women and people of colour, the disabled and the LGBTQ community, we are gathering, sharing and finding strength and safety in numbers. Our talents of connection, communication and community are finding outlets in increasingly creative ways. We are rebuilding networks and rekindling pride in our motherhood.

In my corner of the world a lot of positive work is going on. Women are beginning to gather – an activity that is inherently political, given that gatherings of women have been illegal or discouraged in many cultures for much of human history, most notably in recent years by the Taliban, but also by the Trump administration, which attempted to restrict the Women's March the day after the inauguration. But put 'women gathering' into Google and the list is heartening: red tents, positive birth groups, doulas, online support groups, feminist activists; religious and secular, trans, gay, straight, queer, women of colour – we are coming together. Yes, we argue, sometimes spectacularly, but we are having conversations, learning from each other, working to find a way forward, striving to describe a world where we are all recognised for the contributions we make.

'I spent my teens and early twenties stuck in the patriarchal model that "women are bitchy". In my thirties I really discovered and embraced sisterhood. I have this deep longing/need inside for sitting in circles with women: it fills my soul,

and nourishes me in ways that I find difficult to describe. I feel very blessed to be able to sit with like-minded women like this.'
Sophie Messager

I am imagining. At least, I am trying to imagine a world where women, mothers in particular, are given a voice. Listening to Sandy Toksvig talk about the birth of the Women's Equality Party is illuminating: finding out that only seven FTSE 100 companies are run by women was not what astounded her, it was learning that 17 of them were run by a man called John. Humorous and ironic as that is, I waited in vain for the next point: how many of those seven women are mothers? And why do we spend time talking about glass ceilings, when those in the basement are the ones who need the biggest hand up?

So I am imagining something different: not just more women in business and politics and media and sport, although all these things are important. I'm dreaming of a world where mothers are put at the centre. You see, an infant's relationship with their mother is the primary relationship, the one on which all other relationships and interactions are based, for the rest of that person's life. If we nurture and support this primary relationship, so that mothers feel approved of and supported – financially, morally, practically – in the choices they make for themselves and their families, society will begin to change. As psychologist Mia Scotland says:

'the quality of the bond between a baby and its primary caregivers is predictive (on average) of how healthy, both mentally and physically, that baby will grow to be. It's heavy stuff! With the crisis that we have at the moment with anxiety and depression in our society, these are crucial questions that need ongoing, urgent consideration.'

So I invite you to imagine: what would have happened if all the mums had dictated whether or not their sons went off to the trenches of northern France? What if, when the cabinet discussed British defence plans, the ministers had to ask for the views of their mothers? What if urban planners, health service commissioners and public transport providers had to put parents at the centre of their planning and implementation procedures?

What if, instead of maternity being the Cinderella service of the NHS, pregnant people and their partners were put at the centre of health policy in recognition of the fact that the beginning of life is the beginning of health? What if money, resources, and top-level priority were given to birth and postnatal support, so that families could start life together on a firm footing: a foundation of physical and mental health that would last a lifetime and ripple down the generations, saving millions in healthcare costs on the way?

What if, instead of telling us what is good for us and our children, society stopped, pinned back its ears, and listened? The various and diverse voices of women, mothers, fathers, birthing people and parents are important. Their feelings, their needs and their experiences shape not only their own families, but their communities and wider society.

And what if, rather than assuming all parents want nothing more than to work full time and therefore basing all policy decisions on the non-evidence based idea that childcare is good for children, we asked parents how they might like to structure their family lives? How about we actually accept that 'working mothers' have two jobs – the one outside the home and the one that starts the moment she walks through her own front door?

Mother Ellen Thornhill is lucky enough to be able to think laterally and creatively about how she set things up, deciding to get enough domestic help in the house to enable her to spread herself between baby and job. Being liberated enough to be able to be creative and adapt family and work life so everyone is getting both pleasure and financial stability is a privilege most of us don't have.

'We did try having a nanny (lasted 5 days!!), but M wasn't ready and it was a bit of a mess – plus I still had to do all the hard stuff and the nanny got to have all the fun playing with M... We decided rather than "outsource" our childcare, we'd outsource everything else that takes up our time.'

What if we all had equal opportunities to fashion our family lives; sculpting our work inside and outside the home in ways that suit our individual needs? What if we could adapt and change those paradigms as our children grow and our needs, passions and interests change and develop?

What if, for the sake of us all, we all committed to investing in people, whoever they are and however they describe themselves? We are all gardeners of small humans, all mired in playdoh and Roald Dahl and sticky fingers and slow walks collecting sticks and saying hello to cats and snails; all desperately trying to be happy with 'good enough', all battling guilt and exhaustion and worry. Nurturing the next generation is vital work which, as well as being fulfilling, can be mind-numbingly dull, off-the-scale frustrating and bone-achingly tiring. It deserves recognition and reward.

Mothers make an important contribution: we make people. Without us, our species would not only be in decline, but also, without our enormous, all-encompassing, unconditional motherlove, the world would be a cold and dysfunctional place indeed.

I wonder what would happen if, instead of churning out platitudes, withholding benefits from 'non-working' parents and herding all children into McNurseries,* our governments actually stopped for a moment to consider the evidence.

---

* McNursery: my shorthand for chain nurseries, staffed by young people on minimum wage, run on efficiencies and routines rather than love and adventurous exploration. The childcare equivalent of fast food – necessary from time to time, but potentially unhealthy all day every day.

Somewhere along the line they have misinterpreted the need to invest in the first three years as 'separate children from their parents, stuff them full of academic learning and get women back into the office'.

Becca, from Luxembourg, told me that in her home country:

> 'all nursery/preschool education is completely free, and women who choose to stay at home and take a break from the workforce are paid a very substantial allowance from the state to support this. There's a very clear message that it's a valuable role and one that needs to be facilitated. There is also an amazing service (also free) providing emergency childcare in your home for those days when your child is ill but you just have to be at work: you phone them in the morning, and a fully registered and qualified person turns up within an hour to look after your child. Amazing!'

But what happens when we don't sensitively and flexibly support families appropriately? Research[36] has revealed that around 40% of children are not securely attached to a significant adult caregiver. Psychologists define a secure attachment to be when a child shows some distress when a parent leaves, but can compose themselves when the loved one returns. This kind of attachment is formed in the early months of life and is driven by touch and responsive caregiving. Touch is, quite literally, as important as food to a baby, marking the difference between surviving and thriving.

All this seems obvious to most of us – cuddling a baby comes naturally to most people. Yet it is still common for mothers to be entreated to not pick up their baby when they cry. As recently as the 1980s and 1990s there were those who denied that the lack of loving attention and touch given to babies in the Romanian orphanages accounted for the stark differences in their development, compared to babies put in foster care.

However, studies have shown that children who were placed in foster care developed normally compared to children in orphanage care, whose heads were smaller than average. Children in foster care also showed less distress, had better attention spans and a higher IQ on average. Later studies found that the orphanage-raised group was more than twice as likely to develop mental illness, with more than half of inmates going on to be diagnosed with mental illness.

'Scientific experience consistently shows that, in the short term, orphanage placement puts young children at increased risk of serious infectious illness and delayed language development. In the long term, institutionalization in early childhood increases the likelihood that impoverished children will grow into psychiatrically impaired and economically unproductive adults.'[37]

The evidence is clear. Securely attached children grow into well balanced, morally sophisticated, socially cohesive, healthy adults. The work parents do, particularly, in the early months, is crucial. Where it gets frustrating is when this knowledge is used to blame mothers, rather than as proof that mothers and parents in general need solid, targeted, intelligently designed, loving *support*.

Am I naive to believe that if we gave a secure base to all children by providing solid support to parents that the world would change? What if generation after generation was able to grow up with more empathy? What if there were fewer of us with mother/primary caregiver-shaped holes in our hearts? What if every child had enough to eat, and enough love, and was free from fear, with an affectionate family, free from the worst excesses of poverty, with access to an education that allowed the free flow of ideas and the space to find individual talents and passions?

How much hate, trauma and mental illness would we avoid? How many would be saved the torment of abuse and the need for revenge?

Wherever there is suffering, there are mothers working to alleviate it. Wherever there is hunger, mothers are feeding people. Wherever there is injustice, mothers campaign, march and sit in silent solidarity. It is motherhood which makes us shed a tear in empathy with every other mother in the world. It is motherhood which causes us to nurse those who are lost and alone. In an emergency, a mother will put an orphan child to her breast. And where there is tyranny and oppression, mothers stand shoulder to shoulder with women and other oppressed groups and rise up in peaceful protest.

'The memory of childbirth remains with us – unshakeable, unshareable, but never fully expressed' says Sarah Olney, the Liberal Democrat MP, who believes *'We underplay the achievements of mothers'*. In early 2017, she told MPs in the Commons that she felt that getting her daughter to brush her hair was a more noteworthy achievement than her work in Westminster.

It is the possibility of statements like this, by public figures, that gives me a glimmer of hope for the future. The stories of humankind have for too long been told by men. Perhaps it's time, not only for women's stories to be told, but also for us to stand up and tell them ourselves?

'As women around the world struggle to achieve political, social and economic equality, we must reimagine motherhood as not the central core aspect of womanhood, but one of the many potential facets of what make women awesome. It's time.' Katie Hinde, lactation researcher

We will not be silenced. We are rising. Because deep down, everyone knows that mother-centric politics and economics would heal the world. Rather than berate and obliterate the mother-goddess or even blindly worship her, the world would do well to stop, just for a minute, and listen to its mother.

You are are never 'just a mum'. I hear people using this phrase so often and it breaks my heart. You are important. You are creator-CEO of your family. You are the goddess of many hands. Look in the mirror and feel proud, because the act of mothering *matters*.

Mothers Matter by Kati Edwards

If you ever find yourself in the role of a mother
Rest assured, it's a feat like no other!
You'll need patience like never before
To guide, to protect, to build rapport
It's a huge responsibility, our time we must share
Our children need us, they need us right there
They want to be loved and be understood
A beautiful gift for any childhood
They're little people with their own thoughts and feelings
How can we act to enhance the proceedings?
What do they love, what lights them up?
What can we do to fill up their cup?
We must harness our instincts and learn to trust
While setting boundaries that are fair and just
Show ourselves kindness, be our own best friend
Harness the soul voice on whom we can depend.

There's healing required if our own start was smothered
To resolve all the hurt when we've felt unmothered
From broken communities, we can build our tribe
Surrounding ourselves with our own perfect vibe
We can get together and take back what's ours
Sharing our stories and raising the bar
We can nurse in the boardroom
Frequent the Red Tent
Search out our sisters with whom we can vent
And support each other, so we can care
For our precious children who need us there
And care for ourselves, so the love we can scatter
Because children are sacred and mothers matter.

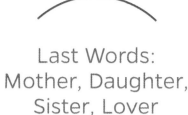

Last Words:
Mother, Daughter,
Sister, Lover

I asked a group of women to write words and phrases that came to mind under the question 'What is a Mother?' The range of ideas and emotions was enormous and the conversation went on long after we had filled the paper and laid down our pens. Each of the words was accompanied by chat, questions, exploration, laughter and tears. What does it mean to you? Could you add to this list? I bet you could.

Something as profound, universal and personal as mothering and motherhood will induce different thoughts and feelings in everyone. Everyone's experience of being mothered and of becoming a parent themselves is unique. All this book could ever hope to do is touch on some of the themes, ask some of the questions and give voices to some 'gardeners of small humans'.

So much of this book has necessarily been about the tough bits, the challenges, the discrimination, the suffering. Yet parenthood can bring a depth of joy that is life-changing, profoundly beautiful and transformative. It has a power to raise us up; it teaches us that there is someone much more important than us. It holds the potential to lift us to a place of wisdom;

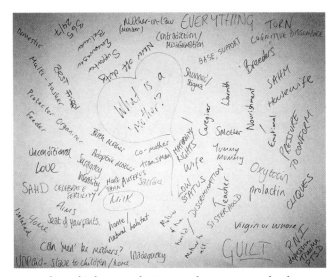

somewhere high enough to see things more clearly – to simultaneously look inward, to our deepest hopes and fears, and beyond ourselves, to view humanity and our future. Spending time with the children you love most in the world can be a transcendent experience. Nothing else has made me so utterly wretched, touched out, furious, frustrated and completely in love and overflowing with bliss in the space of half an hour. In no other job have I ever sat on the toilet seat with the door locked, crying and hiding from screaming children, then been suffused with ecstasy 20 minutes later, lying next to a small, warm person as she nurses to sleep. Breathing out as I trace the perfect line of a cheek with my fingertip, feeling that my heart will burst at the perfection of dark eyelashes resting on flushed silken cheeks.

In no other job have I had the satisfaction of discovering a whole new me. New talents, new capacities and capabilities. My body was never the same again after pregnancy and, for a while, I swallowed whole the message that the new bulges, lumps, saggy bits and stretch marks were ugly and shameful. At first, not feeling attractive, bone-deep fatigue, leaking breasts and the intensity of the trenches of early motherhood took away my libido. I worried sex would never be the same again. I was right, it wasn't. It was better. Eventually.

It is a rarely shared secret that our bodies can work better, be more responsive, more sensitive, more orgasmic after childbirth. And I'm sure age has something to do with it too – women in their 30s are commonly reaching a peak sexually. It does seem that the rush of energy, the euphoria, the sheer primal, animal expression of physicality that is childbirth can sometimes teach women to let go into sexual pleasure in a way that they couldn't access before. Certainly, some women feel they can step into their physicality and more assertively voice their needs after a birth that has felt empowering.

'Sex feels better now. I think physiologically I am the same. Hornier if anything. But I don't know if it's age or the fact that I've done some pretty amazing things with this body, I have more confidence and love for myself now than before.'

'Sex itself is more pleasurable however, as I am more empowered to ask for what I want now, perhaps as a direct result of being so actively involved in my birth choices and taking back my own voice over what happens to my body.'

For some, integrating the dual identities of mother and lover can be tough at first, both emotionally and physically.

'I struggled with the whole Mother/lover dichotomy in the early days, it felt really uncomfortable emotionally and I was very uncertain about what the hell we'd do with these exploding boobs I had!'

For others, the physical manifestations of early motherhood can be hugely erotic:

'There was one occasion, not too many weeks after having my first, when my let-down reflex was triggered at the point of orgasm. We're not talking a dribble either. It was like Niagara Falls coming out of my chest. At first I was mortified but my husband enthusiastically told me he found it totally erotic.'

For many of us, the sheer overwhelming fatigue of the early years has a sobering effect on the libido. For too many, the stresses of becoming a parent put a strain on the relationship or throw existing problems into stark relief. It is still all too common for pain and discomfort during sex to be ignored or considered normal by health professionals and women often swallow the message that they just need to put up with it. Sadly, the 'lie back and think of England' dictat didn't entirely die with the Victorians.

'We tried about three months postpartum but it was really painful and I stopped. I saw the GP about it, then an osteopath. But it took me a while to realise it was because I just didn't want to!'

'I don't think the effect on libido of exhaustion, being touched out and always looking after others gets discussed enough.'

Whether we are talking about sex or any other aspects of ourselves, our identities as mothers will last the rest of our lives. Maybe it's time we stopped metaphorically lying back and thinking of England and started expressing our needs a little more. Because mothers who are fulfilled and satisfied, who feel nurtured and heard, are strong and capable. And strong, capable mothers have love, time and energy to spare – for their partners, their children and their communities. What kind of experience do we want for our younger sisters, our daughters and sons when they have children?

We carry our children with us: wherever we go, there is a room in our hearts for each one of them. Our bodies and minds may change, with time and circumstances; a wild ride of highs and lows and new territories to explore, but the mother-you is always with you. If you're just starting out on your parenting journey, know that your multiple identities will mature. There is no pressure to work out who you are, or what you want. One day, you will be able to look back over the years and survey the landscape of your life; the storms and sunny times, the fertile forest and desert plains, the rivers of tears and the joyful shores, the times of famine and the orchards heavy with the sweet fruit of motherhood. Walking the labyrinth of mothering means inevitably meeting yourself coming back the other way.

Your older self may be grey, but I hope she still has a straight back and a twinkle in her eye, a capacious lap full of grandchildren and passions and pastimes that fire her up. Along the way, I hope she's had lots of women in her life. I hope she had many, many circles of sisters to laugh and cry with through the years. I hope she can peer up her maternal line to her mother, her grandmother and her great-grandmother and see the strong women who spawned her, feel their warm, work-worn hands and hear their words of wisdom.

If you are tending to the next generation, hats off to you. It's a hard, relentless, dirty job. Knee deep in bodily fluids, Lego and guilt, you are the hidden heroes. If you want to work, but can't afford childcare. If you wish you could stay at home with the children, but can't afford to jack in the job. If he's hitting you or emotionally abusing you. If you were raped. If people jump to conclusions about you because of the colour of your skin or who you love. If he gives you 'pocket money'. If you are living in poverty. If you are homeless. If you are running from war or terror. If you are afraid. If your birth rights were ignored.

If you are differently abled. If you are in mental distress of any kind. If your desire to breast or chest feed was sabotaged or unsupported. If you are discriminated against for any reason. If you are criticised for being too young or too old. If you are alone. If you are lonely. If you are bored. If you love every second of it. If mothering is a tiny bit of you, or your whole, blissful world. If they are grown and flown, or you are just starting out with a newborn. If you yearn for kids and can't have them, or wish you didn't have to have any more. If your child died. If your child is sick or has special needs. If you are a surrogate mother or an adoptive mother. If you are raising or helping to raise your grandkids. You are all amazing. You are all doing your best. You are all worthy and wonderful and full of power and potential. This book is for all of you – however you mother, however you were mothered, whoever you are. This is a hymn of praise to the wise women, the warrior women. I bow down before you. You make the world go round.

'Loving myself as a mother is an act of resistance! It's powerful... all of society's ingrained disrespect for women and mothers, double standards, micro-aggressions and even outright aggression. But the more I can love and value myself as mother and love the mothers I work with as a doula, the more light we collectively create. It's really cool.' Aimee Hamblyn

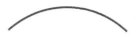

Further Reading

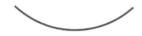

Liberating Motherhood: Birthing the Purplestockings Movement by Vanessa Olorenshaw

What Mothers Do: Especially when it looks like nothing by Naomi Stadlen

The Mommy Brain: How Motherhood Makes Us Smarter by Katherine Ellison

Why Love Matters: How affection shapes a baby's brain by Sue Gerhardt

Musings on Mothering, edited by Teika Bellamy

Of Woman Born: Motherhood as Experience and Institution by Adrienne Rich

Kiss Me!: How to Raise Your Children with Love by Carlos González

The Mother of All Questions: Further Feminisms by Rebecca Solnit

Nobody Told Me: Poetry and Parenthood by Hollie McNish

The Motherhood Constellation: A Unified View of Parent-Infant Psychotherapy by Daniel N. Stern

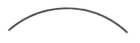

References

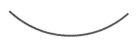

1. www.nysun.com/arts/reconsiderations-betty-friedans-the-feminine/86003
2. onlinelibrary.wiley.com/doi/abs/10.1002/imhj.21527
3. onlinelibrary.wiley.com/doi/abs/10.1111/j.1467-8624.1994.tb00828.x
4. www.npeu.ox.ac.uk/birthplace
5. www.livescience.com/47298-babies-amazing-brain-growth.html
6. thebirthhub.co.uk/2015/07/27/the-whos-who-of-breastfeeding
7. www.sciencenews.org/blog/growth-curve/backwash-nursing-babies-may-trigger-infection-fighters
8. www.ons.gov.uk/peoplepopulationandcommunity/healthandsocialcare/causesofdeath/bulletins/pregnancyandethnicfactorsinfluencingbirthsandinfantmortality/2015-10-14
9. www.maternityworldwide.org/what-we-do/three-delays-model
10. ibid
11. whiteribbonalliance.org/campaigns2/respectful-maternity-care/
12. www.npeu.ox.ac.uk/mbrrace-uk
13. www.nmc.org.uk/about-us/our-role
14. www.guttmacher.org/news-release/2015/teen-pregnancy-rates-declined-many-countries-between-mid-1990s-and-2011
15. www.ncbi.nlm.nih.gov/pmc/articles/PMC2812877/
16. The Risks of Not Breastfeeding for Mothers and Infants Rev Obstet

Gynecol. 2009 Fall; 2(4): 222–231.

17. www.who.int/mental_health/maternal-child/maternal_mental_health/en

18. www.who.int/mental_health/prevention/suicide/Perinatal_depression_mmh_final.pdf

19. www.who.int/mediacentre/factsheets/fs348/en

20. webarchive.nationalarchives.gov.uk/20160105160709/http://www.ons.gov.uk/ons/dcp171776_234036.pdf

21. www.gottman.com/blog/the-research-the-still-face-experiment/

22. adc.bmj.com/content/early/2014/11/12/archdischild-2014-306701.full?g=w_ep_open_tab#block-system-main accessed 12/2/17

23. www.ncbi.nlm.nih.gov/pubmed/7503208

24. internationalbreastfeedingjournal.biomedcentral.com/articles/10.1186/s13006-016-0097-2

25. blackwomendobreastfeed.org

26. ourworldindata.org/a-history-of-global-living-conditions-in-5-charts

27. hilaryburrage.com/fgm and www.dofeve.org/about-us.html

28. www.malala.org/girls-education

29. www.aims.org.uk and whiteribbonalliance.org

30. redtenttemplemovement.com and www.positivebirthmovement.org

31. www.birthrights.org.uk

32. www.birthcompanions.org.uk

33. matexp.org.uk

34. thinkprogress.org/meet-the-people-who-provide-protection-at-abortion-clinics-38f23738547b

35. bmcpregnancychildbirth.biomedcentral.com/articles/10.1186/1471-2393-13-196

36. www.npeu.ox.ac.uk/prumhc/maternity-care-womens-experience-and-outcomes-218

37. www.princeton.edu/news/2014/03/27/four-10-infants-lack-strong-parental-attachments

38. pediatrics.aappublications.org/content/97/4/569.short

Acknowledgements

A book is never the work of just one person so I must acknowledge the immense contributions to the finished product by the following people:

Rachel O'Leary, who lay awake at night thinking of comments and suggestions. Justine Fieth and Verina Henchy, who were my 'book doulas'. Zara De Candole, Zoe Walsh, Nikki Mather, Verity Croft and the other members of my readers' group who challenged, corrected, cajoled and generally carried me through this project. You are my best women and I love you all.

To everyone who so kindly allowed me to quote them, shared their amazing thoughts and stories and allowed me to think out loud online. Special thanks go to the members of the Facebook group 'Feminist Doulas and Midwives', which I started some years ago, but which has grown into the most incredible, safe online space full of the most wise and wonderful birthy people anywhere (yes, I am biased).

A special call out to Vanessa Olorenshaw who first proved to me that I am not alone.

Thanks to Martin at Pinter & Martin, whose quiet faith in my ability to finish and produce something a bit less than disastrous never fails to amaze me. And, of course, quite literally the best editor an aspiring writer could ever hope for – Susan Last, thank you!

Last time I wrote a book my kids were smaller. This time, they hardly noticed but I'll thank them anyway because one day they might actually find it quite cool that their names are in a book or two. So Daniel and Libby, you're always my first inspiration and the reason I do what I do.

And lastly, to the man the doula world calls 'Mr Maddie': thank you for the websites, the patience, the acceptance of all the hours writing instead of being out earning a living. Chris, you're the tops.

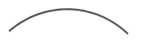

Index

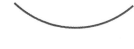

Series editor: Susan Last

pinterandmartin.com